PRAISE FOR GUNNAR PETERSON

"What I once saw to be a tedious, vain endeavor, Gunnar has shown to be a complex science that has positively affected every area of my life."
—DEBRA MESSING

"Gunnar's program is the best and most intense I have ever used. It's the kind that separates the champions from the contenders."
—VERNON FORREST, THREE-TIME WORLD WELTERWEIGHT BOXING CHAMPION

"Gunnar is the only person who has gotten me off my butt and excited about working out. That's a miracle!"
—MICHELLE BRANCH

"Gunnar has exceptional knowledge and motivation when it comes to personal health and fitness. He was extremely beneficial to me and my preparation as an NFL quarterback."
—JEFF GARCIA, CLEVELAND BROWNS

"With G, I've literally laughed my way into the best shape of my life! Thanks, Gunnar—I love you!"
—AMBER VALLETTA

"Gunnar trains every hour like it's the first of the day."
—GARRETT HEDLUND

"In the past, I never really enjoyed working with weights. Now, after three months with Gunnar, I'm addicted!"
—MARKO JARIC, LOS ANGELES CLIPPERS

"I walk in, do five crunches, and eat a Luna Bar. . . . Gunnar has changed my life!"
—DAVID SPADE

"Gunnar Peterson trains the stars, and I train Gunnar Peterson. Trust me, he knows what he's talking about!"
—JON LOVITZ

"When I first heard about Gunnar, a trainer to the stars, I wasn't quite sure how he could relate to a pro athlete. I gained a whole new respect for his expertise when I discovered the rest of his client list, including Pete Sampras, a legend whom I have always admired. One brief phone call before our meeting was all Gunnar needed to put together a killer routine! He combined a sport-specific exercise with a fun, challenging workout, and his knowledge, enthusiasm, and work ethic put him at the top of his field."
—ERIC WEINRICH, PHILADELPHIA FLYERS

"Gunnar's a great guy who does a great job, and he's probably the craziest out there. Keep getting the job done!"
—COREY MAGGETTE, LOS ANGELES CLIPPERS

"Gunnar has changed my views on working out and strength training. Not only am I in the physical shape that I'd always hoped to be, but on a larger scale, training with him has helped me become the kind of person I've always wanted to be."
—SCOTT FOLEY

"In my profession and in my personal life, I always want to be around creative, passionate and energetic people—and there is no doubt that Gunnar possesses all of those qualities. I have loved getting to know Gunnar over the last several years and I really respect his ability to translate those special qualities into teaching people to take better care of their bodies and to believe they can do anything."
—COACH MIKE KRZYZEWSKI, DUKE UNIVERSITY

"I love working with Gunnar. The energy of his gym always makes you want to go back. He has a great work technique that is always fun."
—PENÉLOPE CRUZ

"Gunnar is the best at getting me in the best shape in the least amount of time and the minimum amount of pain. I don't ever dread going to the gym because the day before killed me. . . . On the contrary, I love going because I know I am going to achieve incredible results. With Gunnar, every minute is doing something great for my body."
—JENNIFER LOPEZ

"Gunnar trains my wife Kris and me, but had he trained me for the Olympics in 1976, I would have scored over 9,000 points in the Decathlon. I have been in the fitness business all my life, and there is *nobody* better than Gunnar. He brings out your best possible performance with his passion, work ethic, motivation, and talent . . . and takes fitness to a whole new stratosphere. Gunnar is absolute *gold*."
—BRUCE JENNER

"My experience at Gunnar's gym has been a lot of fun, especially for someone like me who doesn't like gyms. Gunnar's training is challenging and very thorough, and he is unusually focused on each person's particular physical need, whether they are professional athletes, actors, or musicians like me. I would definitely recommend Gunnar to anybody who wants a totally comprehensive workout."
—SLASH

"I had read a lot about Gunnar's star-studded clientele, but it wasn't until I started working out with him that I realized there was a reason his clients raved about him and their results. I had given up on ever enjoying working out, but with Gunnar's positive attitude I actually found myself looking forward to our sessions—and I found myself back in my old jeans in six weeks."
—JULES ASNER

GUNNAR PETERSON

WITH MYATT MURPHY

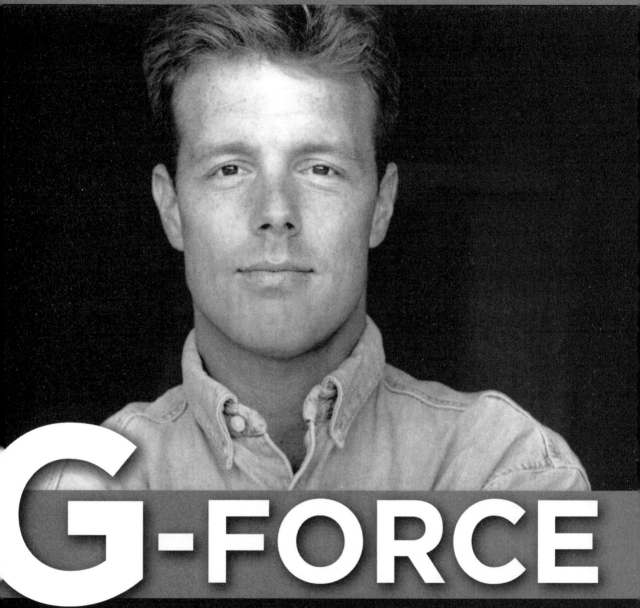

G-FORCE

THE *ULTIMATE* GUIDE TO YOUR *BEST BODY* EVER

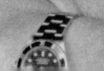 ReganBooks
Celebrating Ten Bestselling Years
An Imprint of HarperCollinsPublishers

Illustrations courtesy of Scott Dalrymple.

All exercise photography courtesy of Mike Lohr, www.MichaelLohrPhotography.com

G-FORCE. Copyright © 2005 by Gunnar Peterson. All rights reserved. Printed in the United States of America. No part of this book may be used or reproduced in any manner whatsoever without written permission except in the case of brief quotations embodied in critical articles and reviews. For information, address HarperCollins Publishers Inc., 10 East 53rd Street, New York, NY 10022.

HarperCollins books may be purchased for educational, business, or sales promotional use. For information please write: Special Markets Department, HarperCollins Publishers Inc., 10 East 53rd Street, New York, NY 10022.

FIRST EDITION

Designed by Kris Tobiassen

Printed on acid-free paper

Library of Congress Cataloging-in-Publication Data

Peterson, Gunnar.
    G-force : the ultimate guide to your best body ever / Gunnar Peterson.—1st ed.
      p. cm.
    ISBN 0-06-073805-7
    1. Physical fitness. I. Title.

RA781.P49 2005
613.7—dc22   2004061351

05 06 07 08 09 RRD 10 9 8 7 6 5 4 3 2

TO EVERYONE WHO HAS EVER
WORKED OUT WITH ME,
THANK YOU.
REALLY, THANK YOU.
SERIOUSLY, I MEAN IT.
THANK YOU.
LISTEN TO ME, WILL YOU?
JUST SHUT YOUR PIE HOLE
AND LISTEN UP FOR ONE
SECOND . . .
THANK YOU!

CONTENTS

INTRO-DUCTION

I shyly stood up after the woman announced to the room that I had lost five pounds in the two weeks since the last meeting. There was warm applause. They actually seemed happy for me. Granted, it was an achievement, but I really hadn't done that much. I mean, I just cut out the half-gallon of ice cream that I ate twice a week like clockwork and substituted mustard where I used to eat mayonnaise. You really don't realize how much mayonnaise you eat until you're eating mustard in its place. Still, it was nice to know that I was on the right track and that I had this support system. Even my mom was in the room. But then again, she was the one who encouraged me to join this Weight Watcher's group in Houston, Texas, so she sort of had to be there. She was also my ride. You see, I was only ten years old, and even in Texas I couldn't get a driver's license.

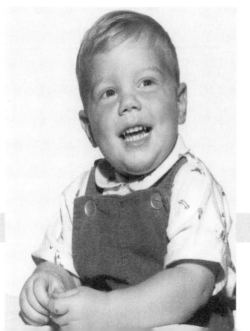

THREE AND TUBBY.

Just to let you know, I didn't continue losing weight at that rate. I started cheating on my diet the very next day at school. I began casually reintroducing two ice cream sandwiches into my regime at lunchtime. Every day. It's not that the ice cream sandwiches were a cardinal sin; it's simply that I was far too young to be morphing into a sneak eater. Believe me when I tell you, old habits die hard (I'm forty-two and I still have the tendencies of a sneak eater).

My childhood in Houston holds many wonderful memories. The formative years often do for people. But weight issues—no matter what age you are—can cast a shadow over even the happiest times, and so not all my memories of growing up are good. Some of my memories come from the back-to-school shopping frenzy that many kids live for. I was no different from other kids in terms of wanting to look "cool," and that meant having the newest, coolest clothes. That was not as easy as it sounds, however, because I couldn't always shop where the other kids shopped. At the time, the big baggy look that today's kids wear was not yet *de rigueur*. Since clothes were a bit more tailored, shall we say, when I was growing up, I had to shop at a special store called Mr. Z's. You know why? Because Mr. Z's carried clothes in "husky" sizes. I cannot begin to describe the shame that made me feel as a kid. Talk about feeling different! For years, I couldn't even look at Husky *dogs*. These shopping trips made quite an impression—evidenced by the fact that some thirty years later, I can still remember the name of the store. I spent every last penny I had at a skateboard store and visited it fifty times a year—compared to my once a year trip to Mr. Z's—but I cannot for the life of me remember *that* store's name. I never had to buy a husky skateboard with special shocks ("trucks" in skateboarding jargon). Coincidence that that shopping experience didn't leave the same kind of lasting mark?

I was sentenced to boarding school in Switzerland at age twelve. In fact, it was more like a five-star hotel than a prison, complete with three square meals a day prepared by an incredible Italian chef, mandatory morning and afternoon teas, and as much pizza and candy as we could make time to eat, not to mention the occasional care package of cookies from friends and family back in the good ol' U.S. of A.

At age fifteen, during the summer, my mother hired a personal trainer for me. I

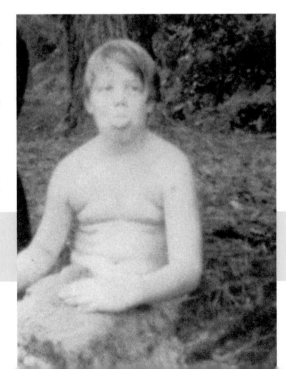

URBANA, VIRGINIA, 1971: AT AGE 9, I HAD JUST WATERSKIED AND NEEDED A BRA . . . OR SHOULD I CALL IT A "BRO"?

went five days a week, alternating weights one day and Chinese Kenpo karate the next. My appointments were at 7 A.M. We were living in Puerto Banus, Spain. Needless to say, this cut into my evening activities quite a bit. At age fifteen in Spain in the summer, there are a lot more things to do than you might imagine. And they're not all healthy. The 7 A.M. sessions probably served more than one purpose in my mother's eyes. While I definitely made progress, it was slowly erased once I was back at school. Still, my interest had been piqued and that turned out to be worth all of those 7 A.M. sessions combined.

I carried my extra pounds (hard to justify it as baby fat when you're twenty-one years old) into and through my college years. At the same time I began taking physical education classes to learn more formally about my burgeoning fitness obsession. I was a walking dichotomy. I worked out fairly regularly. I played sports. And I had my requisite share of college pizza, nachos, and beer—way more than my share of the beer, actually, but that's another book. You see, I was not a complete victim of a poor metabolism, I brought a lot of my weight problems on myself. In fact, we know that very few of us have inalterable metabolic set points. While it may not be easy to change them, these set points are not immovable. It's not that you've necessarily been dealt a bad hand; it's that you may have been playing it wrong over the years and now you have to pay up.

In addition to all of my various activities, healthy and otherwise, I tried almost every diet under the sun except, perhaps, for the Beverly Hills Diet, which involved eating some insane amount of pineapple several times a day. Not exactly convenient. Not exactly easy to fit into the average lifestyle unless you happened to be a cast member of *Gilligan's Island*, *Fantasy Island*, or *Magnum P.I.* and have nothing but time and pineapples on your hands. I also had a ringside seat while my mother tried the Beverly Hills Diet for a period of time that was probably much shorter than it seemed. My father cringed the first few times he heard my mother order three consecutive courses of pineapple in a restaurant—in France, of all places. Whether they had it or not, it was an ordeal. More often than not, they didn't have it. And not just in France. This led my mother to import her own pineapple. It became a BYOP party every time we went out to eat. My mother's version of brown-bagging it became the dominant topic of conversation for anyone within three tables. It was the dominant topic of *nonconversation* at our table—the source of much mealtime tension. This tension only encourages bad associations with food and dining. I needed another bad eating association like Tiger Woods needs a golf lesson.

Eventually, that diet along with a slew of others went the way of acid-washed jeans and mullets. No disrespect to David Spade (a.k.a. Joe Dirt)—who trains with me—intended.

Once out of college, I moved to New Orleans, Louisiana, for two years. This was a turning point both mentally and physically for me. I began to focus more and more on exercise, nutrition, health, and fitness. These words, while often used interchangeably, are in fact very different and do not, by definition, overlap. The topics of my reading material gradually narrowed. I began to devour every written word on exercise, training, and diet. Let me tell you, there's a lot more out there than sit-ups, push-ups, and the traditional four food groups. I also exhibited the characteristics of any college graduate left with disposable income in a fun town. New Orleans offers an incredible array of extracurricular activities, not all of which are entirely conducive to optimal health and physical well-being.

I moved to Los Angeles two years later. When I got there I was the stereotypical kid in a candy store, working out at as many different facilities as I could find, taking every possible class, at all possible hours. In essence, I was home. I was not unlike hoards of others who turned up at all these classes and shunned fatty foods like a nun at a keg party. I did notice, however, that many of these regulars, while diligent in their attendance and well-intended in their efforts, were not as educated as they could be about exercise form and performance. Bad form seemed to be rampant, and this included some of the instructors. Nothing that couldn't be corrected, but certainly something that deserved to be addressed.

When I worked out in college with my fraternity brothers who were on the Duke University football team, there was never any question about my strength. It was nonexistent in comparison to theirs. I learned to check my ego at the door early on and to make perfect form on all of my lifts the priority. It's not that I didn't want to compete or show off or challenge them. It just would have been a joke. I still believe to this day that I saved myself a lot of wasted time and probably countless injuries by taking what was in this case the lower road. The easy way, as it were, was the best way. Twenty-three years later, I have yet to burn out on lifting weights, I have no stretch marks, and I've had no lifting-related injuries.

With that in mind, I continued on my path in Los Angeles. I worked out with many lifting partners right up until the point where they didn't show up. One day someone asked if he could work out with me; I asked what time he had in mind. We agreed on a mutual time, and just as we parted he asked what I charged. Charged? I thought he wanted to train *with* me—I didn't know that he wanted me to be his trainer. There was my first client. And so, a career was launched. That was over sixteen years ago. I've trained upward of 50,000 hours since then. And I've enjoyed *every single hour!* Okay, maybe not every single one, but most of them. And that's the only reason I still do this for a living. If I didn't enjoy my work, I'd take my ball and leave the playground. But I don't because I still enjoy it. I've studied too hard and learned too much not to share this with others. I learned by watching and working out with the pros and by watching and working out with the *true* amateurs. You might be surprised at what you can learn from those who know very little. It helped me to divide the "what to do" from the "what *not* to do."

I continued my reading and application of all things health and fitness in the gym and in the kitchen. My existence as a human guinea pig continued based on topical, logical information instead of hokey, gimmicky, faddish, outdated exercise and diet programs of the past. It was then that I began to see tangible results. And they lasted. At first I was skeptical. I figured that my body had gone into some kind of shock during this latest exercise and nutritional transition and would soon return to its normal smooth, definition-lacking, energy-depleted state within a few days. Surprise—it didn't. In fact, as long as I kept eating this way and exercising this way, I could *completely* control how I looked. As a self-admitted control freak, this appealed greatly to me.

What was even more amazing and comforting was that if I strayed, I mean *really strayed*, from this program, once I got back on track I was in charge of how I looked again. After a few straying episodes, I learned that this recapturing of "the body better" took about two days to every one day of straying. This approximation varied depending on the degree of straying, that should be clear, but two to one is fairly accurate to this day for me. For me. Did you get that? It may be different for you, maybe more, maybe less, but you will be able to regain control! Remember that! I also learned through trial and error that doing a little bit of exercise every day was better than a lot only on the day that my subscription to *Muscle and Fitness* arrived. Obviously, you, as I did, will have to have a plan and a program to go with the plan to ensure that each muscle group gets adequate rest and quality fuel in between work bouts. This will vary somewhat by muscle group and even more by individual. Once that's sorted out and you make it as much a part of your daily routine and as unthinkable to blow off as brushing your teeth, you will experience the steady maintainable improvements that I did. I will provide you with a number of different workouts and ways to vary them so that you remain interested and your body continues to respond. This will help you avoid many of the common mistakes that can derail even the most gung-ho of people. I will

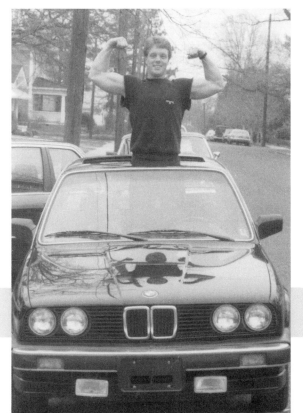

DUKE UNIVERSITY, 1984: JUST GETTING INTO SERIOUS FITNESS. OR SO I THOUGHT.

also share many tips and tidbits that have taken me almost twenty-five years to accumulate, and that may prove to be invaluable to you as you commit to commit! Don't forget, I'm still that chubby little ten-year-old in the Weight Watcher's meeting. I just gathered information and applied it. I had no divine intervention. No burning bush. No celestial openings followed by a Barry White–type voice giving me instruction. I just stuck with it. The password was and is *consistency.*

My experiences, as I pass them on to you, can save you a lot of time and help you avoid a lot of potholes on your road to fitness.

No one *makes* you do anything. *You* are the new sheriff in town. *You* are in charge. So start acting like it. And most of all, have fun along the way.

YOU HAVE EVERYTHING TO GAIN. YOU START EVERY WORKOUT WITH A CLEAN SLATE, EVERY MEAL WITH A CLEAN PLATE. YOU MAKE THE CHOICES. THERE ARE NO VICTIMS.

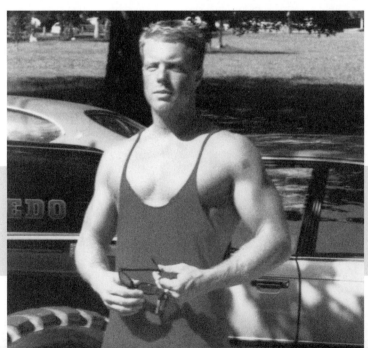

NEW ORLEANS, 1986: BACK IN THE GYM REGULARLY. I DON'T OWN ANY TANK TOPS AND HAVEN'T SINCE THEN, THANK YOU!

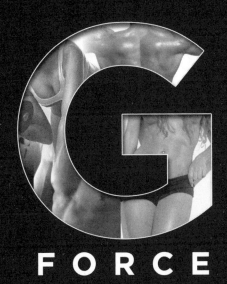

FORCE

PART I

GEAR-
ING UP

Where You Are Now vs. Where You Want to Be

There are three types of people in this world:

1. Those who complain about not being in shape
2. Those who exercise and get in shape
3. And, finally, those who exercise yet still complain about not being in shape

Do you know how many people from category 3 I've met in my life? *Too many* is the answer. Are you that person? If you are, don't worry—we're going to tackle that!

Are you the woman who has endured endless hours of sweat, pain, and cheesy music in countless group exercise classes? The one who's dropped hundreds of dollars on fancy classes—without dropping any weight? Or maybe you're the guy who's been hitting the weights regularly, yet, for some reason, can't get your muscles to grow and get stronger the way they used to. It's a classic story with the same sad ending. In short, a certain exercise routine worked for you at one time, but now it just isn't cutting it like it used to.

How you approach your exercise is often as important as how often you exercise. It doesn't matter if you're the most devout gym rat in your neighborhood and haven't missed a day of exercise since gas was a dollar a gallon. You may still be a victim of poor exercise habits without realizing it.

Are you known as the "cycling nut" or a "die-hard runner" at work or among your friends? Or are you a blur in the gym, popping from machine to machine without any rhyme or reason—not bothering to keep track of anything that you've done?

Maybe you're the type who's tried every class, every machine, and every exercise imaginable. You've never grown tired of pushing yourself as hard as you can, as often as you can—much to the amazement of the general public who probably looks at your commitment as a sign of insanity.

Or are you the exact opposite? The type who finds it hard to get motivated at the gym? The beginner who wants to exercise, but feels intimidated by the equipment and/or the people around that equipment? Or could you be the perpetual off-and-on exerciser? One month, you're hard at work in the gym. The next month, you're hardly breaking a sweat. You're the exerciser who dedicates yourself to getting fit only when it fits in with your life.

Do you know why I know all these personalities like the back of my hand? Because I've trained each and every one of them! I know what it takes to drive you to exercise year-round, but I also know that you've got to be careful or that same driver will eventually demonstrate the skills of a crash test dummy. You've got to be smarter about what you're doing as you proceed if you want to continue to see progress.

So, which type are you?

Guess what? It doesn't matter anymore. No matter what type of person you are in this world, no matter what type of personality you are, I've got the solution to getting you in the best shape ever. It's a little thing I call *G-Force*. So if you're ready, let me introduce you to the four words that will change your life.

The Four F-Words

It's not easy staying in shape when you're as busy as you are, right? I know. Trust me, I know.

You spend your workday, well, working. You probably spend the bulk of it trying to satisfy a demanding boss or getting through a tough workload. During your off-hours and weekends, you're trying to make the most of time with loved ones. You've got 48,000 errands, responsibilities, and obligations filling in the cracks of your leisure time. So when you finally find a free minute to yourself in all that chaos, all you want to do is relax. Often, that means an activity that barely requires a pulse! It's no wonder that exercise and fitness get pushed to the bottom of your personal list.

I don't care whether you were once in amazing shape or have never exercised at all. You've turned to me because you're fed up with where you are now. You're turning to me just like my clients did when they decided that their bodies needed to look and function better. I'm glad you're here, because being here is going to make what I have to tell you that much easier to understand. Being here is the first step to getting *there*.

Let me guess: You think that not having enough time to devote to exercise is your only problem. I know what a busy lifestyle is all about because everyone I work with deals with that very same issue. *I* deal with that same issue! I understand how inconvenient and futile exercise can seem when every possible problem in life is demanding all of your attention and your time. But I have good news and bad news for you:

LACK OF TIME IS ONLY ONE PIECE OF A MUCH BIGGER PROBLEM.

Whenever someone I used to work with comes back looking like they not only fell off the wagon but ate the horse that was pulling it, I know they've dropped the ball on one of the four "F-words":

1. Function
2. Foundation
3. Freedom
4. Focus

These F-words are the reason you're swearing at yourself in the first place. C'mon now, you know what word comes to mind when you step on the scale and see a number blinking up at you that looks more like a high bowling score than your actual weight. Seriously, what word pops into your brain when you try slipping into an old pair of pants and you end up ripping into them instead? You know there's some not-acceptable-for-network-television expletive hanging off the tip of your tongue whenever you see someone older than you looking younger and fitter than you!

You're angry.
You're fed up.
You're frustrated.
Well, guess what?
You should be.

From now on, every time you think, say, or scream anything foul because you don't look the way you want to look, you're going to remember why you're fed up in the first place. So go ahead, swear all you want. Pick a body part and unload on it with a mouth that would earn you the "bar o' soap" lunch special when you were a kid. Stare at that old belt that looks like it was washed in hot water. Now, take those thoughts and that energy and turn it around. We are going to use those feelings to get you on track and keep you on track.

It doesn't matter whether you're struggling to take off twenty pounds of stubborn fat, desperate to put on ten pounds of eye-popping muscle, or just hoping to be in decent enough shape to walk your dog without wheezing all the way up the block. You need to get the four F-words under control, and you need to do it now.

Let's take a closer look at how the F-words have been derailing the results you deserve.

FUNCTION

Being a certified fitness professional gives me *carte blanche* to get my clients to do anything I want them to do.

I'm talking anything here.

I can completely ruin their world by telling them we're trying something new today. I could make them grab a dumbbell with one hand and a half-filled glass of water in the other. Then, I could tell them to stand on one foot in the most painfully awkward position I can dream up. Finally, just to make things more entertaining, I could have them spell out their middle name in the air twelve times with each elbow. Watching them shake around, getting soaked like they're having a grand mal seizure on a water ride, may make me sound like a sadist (I've been called worse!), but it's just my little way of making a serious point.

Do you ever, and I mean *ever*, do anything important without investigating it first? Would you plunk down all your hard-earned dough in the stock market without knowing a single thing about the companies you're about to invest in? Okay, bad example. I mean, would you plunk down all your hard-earned dough in the stock market without knowing a single thing about the companies you're about to invest in, *again*? Would you stick your kids in a daycare center that contacted you without checking to make sure the owners don't have their "headshots" pasted on post office walls nationwide? Of course not! So why would you obediently do what you're told when it comes to exercise without questioning why you're doing it? By questioning, I don't necessarily mean disputing. I just mean asking. Informing yourself. Just like anything else.

Fitness failures can't answer me if I ask them, "Do you know why you're doing that movement?" Oh sure, they may confidently spit out whatever body part that exercise is working, but they have no idea what that exercise is actually *doing* or if they're truly using good form. Most people exercise like babies, copying what they see others doing, but lacking a clue about why they're doing it in the first place.

Having no sense of function brings a host of problems to the fitness failure's workout. It can have you working muscles in the wrong order or in an ineffective order, which often results in tiring out smaller muscles too quickly before the larger ones you're trying to work get enough of a workout. This sequence can lead you to unintentionally overwork certain muscles and connective tissue—especially around the shoulders, elbows, and knees—to the point of diminishing returns or worse, injury. It can leave you ignoring muscles that desperately need your attention. In short, it can keep you from unveiling your best you.

You need to be educated in every facet of exercise so you can make it work for you and not against you. Every chapter of *G-Force* is designed to do exactly that, which is why it's crucial that you read every chapter as seriously as the rest. That way, you'll finally learn how to work out in order to accomplish what you're hoping to accomplish. After all, you're the one who's ready to dedicate countless hours to exercise in order to get in some kind of shape. Do you really want someone having you do something wrong or, God forbid, something that would make you look foolish because you didn't know the difference?

I didn't think so.

FOUNDATION

Would you sign up for a marathon if you had never run a day in your life? Would you apply to college if you hadn't taken the SAT? C'mon, these are no-brainers. So how can you expect to succeed in fitness when you haven't even bothered learning a few of the most basic tenets?

FOUNDATION = TIME + BASICS + PLAN + FUEL

Not Locking in Enough Time

Fitness failures don't take exercise seriously enough to budget adequate time for their workouts. I'm not just talking about the half hour or hour you plan to work out; I'm talking about making sure you have enough time for all the minutia you have to do before and after your exercise.

After all, it's the things you're doing right before you exercise and the things you're doing right after that eat into your workout time. The fitness failure doesn't budget enough time to get to the gym, change into workout clothes, warm up, work out, and clean up afterward.

Answer me this: You're in the middle of your workout and realize you've got an urgent meeting that you must attend. Do you finish your workout, skip a shower, and go back to your office smelling like a longshoreman? Or do you skip the last few minutes of your workout to get scrubbed up? Please, I have my answer. And I hope you have yours. Not offending your colleagues with your o-dear is an important priority, but it proves that if you don't plan in advance, your workout will always get shorted.

It's like going to a play late, catching only the second act while feverishly checking your watch, then having to leave before finding out if the guy gets the girl, not to mention missing the fat lady's song. Did you go to the play? Yes, technically you did. Did you get as much from it as the person who showed up early, read the playbill, and sat through the whole thing? No! That's why it's critical to give yourself the block of time it takes to get there, park, get in there, get it done, get out, get cleaned up, and get back to wherever you have to be. If you don't have that block built into your foundation, you're behind before you start.

Not Locking Down the Basics

Too many people feel enticed to try whatever fancy move they read about in the latest issue of their favorite fitness magazine. Now don't get me wrong: I'm a big believer in many of those quirky, off-the-wall exercises. I'd be a hypocrite if I weren't a fan, because sometimes it's even my version of the exercise that is being featured! The thing to remember is that no matter how original an exercise may seem, chances are, it's just one of a hundred variations of a basic exercise you should have learned and spent time doing first!

Each workout is just one brick in your foundation. Sticking to the basic exercises, which I'll walk through with you, and learning how to do them with *perfect* form is all anyone ever needs to start reshaping himself and to avoid injury. Fitness failures forget that point and throw all their energy into the most advanced exercises they've read about or seen someone in better shape do in their gym. That's like picking out the fastest car in the lot before you learn how to drive. It's also why those exercises either leave you in pain later or never really seem to work—a lot like having an accident in that fast car.

Not Locking Down a Plan

If you came to me to work with you, how would you feel if you showed up at my gym and I had no plan for what I was going to do with you that day? Well, imagine how your body feels every time you give it that same "I'll figure it out as I go along" approach. Just showing up doesn't cut it. It's how well you prepare for exercise that ultimately determines what you're going to get out of the exercise.

Fitness failures head to the gym with absolutely no game plan. They don't bring a sheet of paper that tells them what they're going to do that day, either because they don't know what to write, feel too self-conscious to look at it during their workouts, or think they just don't have the time. If I timed you, it would probably take you less than five minutes to get everything you actually needed down on paper.

Five minutes.

Locking down a plan doesn't have to be some long, drawn-out painful process that makes you wish you were someplace or someone else. It's a simple checklist that runs down what you are planning to do that day regarding your workout. You could do it over breakfast (the meal you're going to start eating). You could do it over lunch. You could do it while listening on the phone to your mom talking about the latest thing that grew on her foot. The point is, writing down what you need to do is as essential as bringing a map with you on a long drive. Without any directions, it's easy to lose sight of your destination.

Writing down your plan isn't just about tracking your progress. Not doing it also cheats you of feeling any sense of accomplishment. Without a plan, you can't cross the word *exercise* off your "stuff I had to do today" list. Here's a rule to remember:

KNOWING YOU HAD A PLAN, STUCK WITH IT, AND COMPLETED IT IS ONE OF THE GREATEST MOTIVATIONAL TOOLS EVER.

I promise you, just get through one week, and you'll be inspired to stay on track the next week. The sense of accomplishment will fuel your desire for more accomplishment. In my sixteen-plus years as a trainer, I've never seen this *not* happen with a client. That's what it takes on a day-to-day, week-to-week, month-to-month, year-to-year basis to stay the course. I believe in this rule so strongly that whenever new clients who are fired up to train with me want to start by doing it every day, I try to rein it in a bit without curbing their enthusiasm, and set them on a more realistic approach.

For example, I'd rather have my clients book two workouts for the week, show up for those two, get the work done in those two, and know that they did what they set out to do. If I can't convince them to do it that way, what inevitably happens is they'll book three or more workouts, cancel one *or more*, beat themselves up for what they *didn't* do, and deny themselves credit for what they did do. Eventually, they quit because all they see are the workouts skipped instead of the ones they completed. (Not to mention, the stress from overbooking, canceling, and trying to make it up can create a cortisol buildup in the body. Cortisol is a hormone that your body produces when it is under stress, and it's been proven to make the body more likely to retain body fat. Needless to say, from a fitness standpoint, cortisol is not your friend.)

Not Locking Down Your Fuel

You can't drive a race car without putting any gas in it. Over time, you'd be lucky if it even started! I keep an assortment of energy and protein bars and performance drinks (like Gatorade) in my gym. Even the most discriminating palate can find something here! I do this because I understand what happens in the life of a busy person. Time just gets away from you. And I know that if someone comes to me on an empty gas tank, the hour I'll spend working with him or her is not going to be optimal for either of us.

Too often, it's the people who are concerned with burning calories who forget to take them in before their workout. Starving yourself is not the answer to reaching your goals. If there's nothing in your body to allow your muscles to work, you're done before you even begin. If you're the fitness failure who wakes up, slaps on your running shoes, and hits the pavement with nothing in your stomach in an effort to burn more body fat, you've missed the part about how nutrition and exercise work hand in hand. Read the chapter about food and exercise closely!

FREEDOM

Do you know why so many people are stowing away on boats, running across patrolled borders under the cover of darkness, or huddling in the back of an old truck sitting on the floor with thirty other people just to get to America? Because they see this country as the land of opportunity—a place where, if you have a dream, no matter how noble, ambitious, or slightly disturbing it might be, you stand the best chance of making that dream a reality because of the freedoms we have here. Having freedom means having choices. The more freedom you have, the more choices you have, period.

My mom always told me that only the boring are bored. It's a piece of wisdom that carries itself right into exercise. Remember when I said it was crucial to have a plan and stick to it? Well, being able to modify that plan into a new routine when it becomes too boring or less effective is still part of that plan. When it comes to working out, your exercise options are endless. I know, because it's my job to whip up all of those options. I'm up between 3 A.M. and 4 A.M. every day changing the exercises, the sets, the reps, the sequence, the intensity, the duration, and more in every client's routine. My goal is that they never, ever do the same workout twice. Most people have no idea how to do this for themselves because they're not aware of just how much freedom they have with exercise. Fitness failures know only a handful of exercises. It's usually some old routine they've been carrying around with them since they had a hairline *and* a waistline. But now the same routine that may have worked back then has become outdated and close to worthless to them in their current physical condition.

So maybe your old back can't handle the same workout you used to do in your twenties. Figuring out what exercises may be smarter to use now—rather than rigidly sticking to what may have worked in the past—takes just a nominal amount of common sense that most people lack. Not knowing how to modify an exercise to make it more effective leaves you feeling powerless and trapped. It prevents you from moving from station to station, exercise to exercise, machine to machine, without always having to stop or slow down your workout just to think about what to do next. It deprives you of enjoying every single workout because you're always limited while exploring new ways of getting in shape.

Lack of freedom—being too rigid in your routine—also makes it harder to stand up and accept adversity in your workouts. The fact that you may know all of the steps necessary to get yourself to go from point A to point B doesn't mean that road is a journey without obstacles and moments of failure. Life has a way of throwing a few surprises into everyone's workout, usually in the form of some knucklehead who won't get off the machine you need to use next, or worse, won't *wipe* it off. If you aren't adept at changing your workouts in a pinch around any negative encounters that may interfere with your goals, you're on a one-way street instead of an eight-lane highway.

Fitness failures never have what I call an "exercise contingency plan." What would you do if you suddenly had only thirty minutes to exercise instead of sixty minutes? What if a meeting or appointment ran late and you didn't get to eat beforehand so that you were too hungry to exercise, or if you were too tired to exercise because you had not eaten? Lacking freedom makes it harder to prevent all the things that have ever derailed you from fitness. Having freedom means you'll be battle-ready for every emergency situation that's ever poked a hole in your plans because if it's ruined your workouts before, trust me, it could ruin them again.

Finally, freedom keeps the results from stopping. Sticking with certain exercises or activities is fine, if that's what gets you results. However, your body learns to adapt quickly to constant stress. Keep repeating "any" exercise or activity and your body eventually wises up and discovers an easier way to get the same job done using fewer muscles and burning fewer calories. That's why you're leaving the gym tired from exercising but more exhausted from never seeing anything improve.

Why else does that suck? Sticking with one exercise can overwork certain muscles while ignoring others, which will keep you from achieving the perfect shape you're looking for (unless you really want to look like a walking funhouse mirror). And if that doesn't scare you, then maybe this will. As any muscle gets stronger, it begins to pull on the opposing muscles behind it. When there is an imbalance in the strength of those opposing muscles and they are too weak to resist, they can be pulled or strained more easily. Or even worse, they can cause certain joints, like your elbows, shoulders, and knees to shift out of alignment. Not a good look.

Finally, having freedom lets you mix it the f@*# up!!! That should get your attention.

I'm saving my real "F-word" allowance for later! If this is all you take away from this book, you will improve—so go for it. You won't have to give up whatever gets you into exercise, but for God's sake, you need to change how you do it every once in a while. There are three components (frequency, intensity, and time) that you can adjust with any and every exercise, whether you're addicted to cardiovascular training or weight training. The **frequency** is how often you exercise, or how often you target a specific body part. The **intensity** is how fast you perform the exercise or how much weight you use. The **time** is how long your workout lasts or when you work out. Changing just a few or all of these factors every six to eight workouts can turn that same boring exercise that others would hang themselves doing all the time into a new challenge for your body.

FOCUS

Once you know why you're exercising in the first place (Function), all the basics (Foundation), and how to change things around so you're never at a loss to surprise your muscles ever again (Freedom), you're not done yet because you still need to know how to focus on exercise.

The fitness failure goes through the motions, never giving exercise 100 percent of the attention it deserves. It's like going to lunch with a friend you haven't seen in years, who then spends the whole meal yapping on his cell phone. Your friend actually believes he's caught up with you, while simultaneously listening to whoever's talking to him on the phone. But all he's really managed to do is ruin a potentially good time and use valuable minutes on his calling plan.

In the busy lives we lead, multitasking takes over every hour of the day, including sleeping! How many "Lose weight while you sleep" or "Make money while you sleep" ads have you seen? But you need to shut it out of your workout if you want to see the results you crave. You may be focused during certain parts of your routine, but if you're not focused throughout each and every step, you're not getting the most out of your time. Whenever you "phone in" any portion of your workout, you make it less effective than it could have been. Did you spend twenty minutes on that stationary bike? Sure, your behind remembers being planted on that uncomfortable seat, but if your brain isn't concentrating on the ride because you were too busy reading the personal ads or doing the crossword puzzle, your body ends up spending less energy and getting fewer results because *you* tuned out. Sure, you did something. But you didn't do it as well as you could have.

Not Focusing on Your Body

Sorry, but just showing up to work out doesn't cut it.

I've had clients who thought that because I've worked with athletes, actors, and actresses who got in fantastic shape the same thing would instantly happen to them after they decided to train with me and showed up for one or two workouts. *News flash*: It doesn't work that way. For some, this was a wake-up call as to how hard they were going to be pushed to get them to where they wanted to be. But for you, it's all about pushing yourself as hard as you need to if you want to accomplish these same things.

For the first two years of my working-out life, I never felt the work in the muscles in my back (the latissimus dorsi, or lats). Even after a sixty-minute back workout, I was never really sore in my lats. In fact, it was hard for me to really feel any muscle I couldn't see in the mirror. Not only was I not sore after the workout, but I really wasn't able to feel the contraction in my back *during* the workout. This was not the fault of my program; it was my fault. I didn't know what I was doing or what I was supposed to do.

When I watch someone who is training with me as he is working out, I'm not looking for him to reach any magical numbers or totals with the exercises he's doing with me. I'm looking for only one thing: *effort.*

Did you try? I mean really try? Many people look at exercise as something they can just check off, be done with, and then kick back and reap the rewards afterward. It doesn't work that way. In order to get the most from any exercise, you need to actually feel your muscles flexing as you perform the exercise. If you're not feeling each muscle you're trying to reshape as you're exercising, you're missing out—and your body probably shows it.

Not Focusing on the Movement

Fitness failures plow through workouts like they're late for a wedding—their own wedding. My clients are told all the time that whenever they do an exercise with me, they need to move and think in the same way they would waking up in a strange room that was pitch black. Think about the last time you woke up in an unfamiliar place in the middle of the night. You didn't spring from the bed and charge for the pottie, because you were unfamiliar with the territory. Instead, you moved slowly as you felt around for the light switch, reaching along the walls very carefully so you didn't snap off a fingernail or stub your toe. You became fully aware of where your body was, even though you couldn't see an inch in front of your face. For that one, brief moment, you forgot about your distended bladder and focused on finding just one thing: that damn light switch!

That's how you need to approach every single exercise that you'll eventually use in this book. It's not a race, unless you're competing with all the other overeager exercisers out there to see who can tear a muscle or snap a tendon faster. Trust me, over time, you'll become more proficient and instinctually know where to find that light switch. Eventually, your body will memorize every placement and motion, but that mind/muscle connection will never happen if you never focus on the movement.

Not Focusing on Your Goals

Fitness failures lack focus on having a definable goal to strive for. Having that degree of specificity gives you a road map. It serves as a constant reminder of why you're doing this in the first place. If you're drawing a blank on exactly why you're working out in the first place, or if your reason is something vague, such as "I just want to look better" or "I want to have a better quality of life," you need to go to the blackboard and show your work. Give me some detail. No, let me rephrase that. Give yourself some detail. Dig for a second. It's there.

Maybe your goal is to gain or lose twenty pounds or lower your blood pressure forty points. Those are great goals for different reasons, but they're also big goals that may be hard to swallow in one sitting. I've watched many people over the last sixteen years focus strictly on their long-term goal and fail. Even fail miserably. These people inevitably doom themselves to failure because they are blind to the small, slow, steady accomplishments that, when added up, equal the long-term goal. It's the old "forest for the trees" saying. They are looking so far down the line that they miss the day to day. If you take a page out of John Lennon's book and "enjoy the journey, not just the destination," you'll be better off in the long *and* the short run. Fitness failures don't appreciate how far they have come because they're focused only on the finish line.

Once you have your goals in stone, you need to divide and conquer them. If one of my client's goals is to drop twenty pounds, then I divide that by ten so he has ten smaller short-term goals of losing two pounds each. If his goal is to be able to play basketball for an hour like he did when he was twenty, then I divide that time up by ten so he has ten smaller short-term goals of playing six minutes longer than he did before. Why? Because then he's much more likely to get in and stick with the plan, rather than feel frustrated that he's not attaining his long-term goal, blame it on the workout, and quit.

Not Focusing on Reality

I work with some of the world's greatest athletes—individuals who redefine just how far the human body can be pushed. But I have news for you that some of these stellar athletes may not fess up to publicly: Even *they* have their off days.

Fitness failures beat themselves up over the things that sometimes just can't be helped. You need to give every workout your best effort, but realize that not every workout is going to be your personal best. Each muscle in your body can have its off days too, which can put a kink in your daily plans for the rest of your body sometimes. That also goes for anything unexpected. I know I told you to make every possible exercise contingency plan, but there will be times when you're faced with the unanticipated, unplanned for, unexpected. If you normally exercise for forty-five minutes, yet have only twenty minutes to give one week because it just ended up that way, then that's what it is and that's fine as long as it doesn't happen regularly. Try to put the extra effort into your food and sleep that week. Make it all work *for* you, not against you.

It doesn't always have to be more.

Sometimes, though, it can be your own fault that you're not living up to your expectations. Are you biting off more than you can chew by using a program you're not ready to use yet? Are you trying to devote more time to fitness than you really can afford to spend? If so, then you need to back off on the demands you put on yourself so you can bump them up later when you're ready to do so. Remember, be consistent and progress.

It's only fitting that the last mistake with which to end this chapter is the one that knocks the most contenders out of the ring. How bad would it suck to know that you might have been well on your way to creating the perfect, Hollywood-honed body, but you gave up too soon?

Being too quick to abandon ship because a plan isn't working fast enough for you is the worst crime you can commit. Fitness failures don't give exercise enough time to do its job, but it's not their fault. Constantly bombarded with every other fitness supplement, product, and book, all touting faster results with less effort, most people doubt they're doing the right thing, especially when their results seem to come more slowly. This brings me to the most important rule in my book:

YOU NEED TO STICK WITH YOUR PLAN LONG ENOUGH TO ALLOW CHANGE TO COME INTO EFFECT. DO NOT LEAVE THE GAME EARLY!

Stop beating yourself up for what you didn't do and start praising yourself for all that you did do.

That last sentence, by the way, should cross over into many aspects of your life if you get what I want you to get out of this book, from fitness to reading, to kids, to marriage, to work, to e-mails. Re-read it and commit it to long-term memory. Ultimately, fitness is about taking the best possible care of yourself, and giving yourself the proper appreciation—instead of constantly tearing yourself down—will allow you to do this. When you start applying the lessons I'm about to teach you, and then stick with them, I promise you, the results will come.

After that, the only F-word coming out of your mouth will be to describe how fantastic you look!

The True Cost of Fitness

Follow the four Fs (Function, Foundation, Freedom, Focus) and you'll be on the road to a whole new you. Now, all you need is the master plan that can take you there. If the four-F plan is the road to perfect fitness, then what you need next is a great car to drive on that road. But before I show you your new ride, let me ask you this: If you're reading this book, then you already know what you want from me, right?

So what is it?

For almost everyone, exercise is simply a means to an end. For some, that end may be losing twenty pounds of fat, while for others that end could be gaining twenty pounds of sheer, rock-hard muscle. Maybe it's to be around long enough to see your great-grandkids being born or just to outlive your third husband. Whatever it is, you need to give yourself an answer and know what you expect from exercise. By the way, there are no wrong answers. No one is judging. You need to have a mental benchmark so that you don't second-guess yourself. Take a second to find your answer. And, no, you don't have to say it out loud.

Is your goal to whittle down that behind, which has recently expanded into a "behind-and-sticking-out-to-the-sides-and-falling-toward-the-floor"? Or could it be to lift fifty more pounds on the bench press to impress your friends? I want you to think about your goal and focus on it as you read this book. That's right. Take a moment to figure out exactly what's going to get you through the journey ahead. Dog-ear this page, and write it here. It's okay, it's your book. Focus on your goal now if you want. I'll wait.

Okay, now that you have it, focus right here at this very page, and I'm going to reveal exactly how to make that specific goal happen just for you. Are you focusing? Hey, if you don't want me to help you out, then that's your . . . ahhhh, there you go!

There's a reason I'm confident that we can get you to that goal. You see, it doesn't matter what your personal, physical, and psychological hopes and dreams are for finally taking exercise seriously. You can't drive toward developing a perfect physique without four wheels.

That's right. I said four wheels, or fitness factors, if you will.

The best-laid fitness plans, and I'm talking about the ones that work 100 percent of the time, must always focus on the following four fitness factors:

1. **Aerobic training** (any activity that elevates your heart rate and maintains that rate for at least 20 minutes)
2. **Resistance training** (any activity involving weights, cables, or any form of resistance that challenges your muscles enough to become stronger and more functional)
3. **Nutrition** (making sure what you eat, drink, or generally stuff into your piehole is working *toward* your goals and not against them)
4. **Rest and recovery** (giving your body enough time to sleep, relax, and recover from your workouts and your life in general)

Each one of these four factors is just as important as the next. Each one deserves the same amount of effort from you at all times. I want you to look at each one as a single wheel on a car. You don't believe it takes all four to drive down the path to a better body? Then I want you to do some thinking for me again. Think back to each and every time you've ever tried to get yourself in shape and didn't succeed. If you can't remember watching your diet, doing both resistance and cardio training, plus being fully aware of how much time your body needed to recover in between, then you already have the answer to why you're still in the same unsatisfying shape. I will bet you the screws in my back that every time you tried to get in shape but fell short of your original goals, it was because you were teetering down the road with one, two, or three wheels, instead of cruising with all four.

I've had muscle-obsessed athletes who thought they were in the best shape of their lives because they lifted weights all the time. They tried driving to a better body by using resistance training only, then wondered why they couldn't increase the weights they used or even run a few blocks without breathing like Pee Wee Herman at the movies. They were only willing to drive on one wheel.

I've watched any number of women who were too paranoid to even consider weight training because they *knew* the secret to dropping fat and feeling great was running more miles every day. In their case, they tried driving to a better body by using aerobic training only, only to end up scratching their heads when their hamstrings or knees gave out after a few months of constant abuse. Again, they were only willing to drive with one wheel.

When I was younger, I watched my mom deprive herself on the latest and greatest diet trends of the times—all of which promised to melt away fat. She tried getting a better body through fad nutrition and spent too many years battling her weight in frustration and without success. She thought that all she needed to do was use one or two wheels (the second being exercise). She finally got it later in life and now looks great, but not until she was willing to drive on all four wheels! Coincidence? You do the math.

And finally, I've watched the rest of the world sit on their bigger and bigger asses every day of the week, week in and week out. They don't exercise. They don't watch what they eat. Whether or not they're aware of it, they're the ones focusing on rest and recovery. And yet they shake their heads in confusion, wondering why they don't have the body they once did. Rest allows the body to recuperate from hard work. But if you're just sacking out on the couch after a sedentary day at the office, the only thing you need a break from is your own lethargy.

I won't deny that you can get certain results from driving on one wheel alone, but you won't get optimal results. Your body is a whole that needs to be trained right, fed right, and rested right. Genetics, good or bad, do only so much for so long. The rest is up to you. And me.

I don't care if running like someone set you on fire or eating lettuce sprinkled with lemon juice has helped you lose weight in the past. I don't care if hoisting weights over your head every single day—without taking time off—has reshaped your physique in the past. And no, I don't care how much you insist you can get by on three hours of sleep and have in the past. I've tried all these things myself and none of them cut it. Eventually, if you're not driving on all four wheels, it's going to take longer for your body to get where it really could go.

Fitness and supplement product companies know that my four-point plan is the key to a better body, but don't count on them to tell it like it is. It's up to you to become a more discerning consumer. Listen closely to almost any infomercial, or squint at the fine print of any pill, product, or miracle-diet book you've ever been suckered into buying. Hidden somewhere, and trust me, it's almost always there, is some disclaimer that covers their behinds—not yours—when their product doesn't work for you. There's usually a line that reads something like, "This product can help you successfully [insert bullshit promise here] when used in conjunction with a sensible reduced calorie diet and regular exercise." What they don't tell you is that if you just watched your diet and exercised regularly without using their product, you'd probably still melt away fat and build muscle to an acceptable degree. The gimmick is just a distraction from what's really reshaping your body. Look, if you need a distraction from the work I'm about show you how to do, then eat a packing peanut every day and call it the "fat-busting wonder snack," if it makes you feel better.

I told you before that I wouldn't have any quick fixes for you. All I have is the truth, and that's what you need to have. If you don't have all four wheels on your car, then put your perfect physique in park because you're not going anywhere. Aerobic training. Resistance training. Nutrition. Rest and Recovery. If you're ready to motor on all four wheels—and get rid of that spare tire at the same time—then it's time to burn rubber.

THE G FORCE PRO- GRAM

The First Wheel: Aerobic Training

This is the wheel that those desperate to lose weight fast always drive on first. Even though it's not the answer to helping you obtain that celebrity-perfect look by itself, aerobic exercise (or cardiovascular exercise) is still a very valuable wheel. Remember that the more you apply yourself to it, the more mileage you'll get from each wheel. Dabbling doesn't work.

THE FACTS

Function

Without aerobic training, you'll lack adequate stamina to push your muscles beyond what they're capable of doing so they will become stronger and shape up faster. Without aerobic training, you'll have to watch calories religiously, which means substituting the foods you actually like to eat with tasteless foods that might not be your first, second, or fiftieth choice. Without aerobic training, your body won't be as efficient at flushing out the toxins that resistance training leaves behind, such as lactic acid (the stuff responsible for creating that fiery, painful, burning sensation that you may experience during and after your workouts). Add the fact that aerobic training improves the quality of your sleep and it's pretty easy to see how it fits into helping you get the most bang from that portion of your proverbial buck.

On its own, it does a lot more than just control and reduce the body fat that's already annoying you. Regular aerobic exercise improves your level of fitness by making your heart stronger so it can work more efficiently. The end results: more oxygen in your system to facilitate physical activity, a reduced risk of depression and anxiety, and an increase of the good cholesterol (HDL) in your system (which has been shown to reduce the risk of heart disease). In fact, your risk of everything, including high blood pressure, stroke, diabetes, and certain types of cancers, such as colon cancer and breast cancer, all decrease as soon as you start sweating a little. And, no, a sauna does not count.

Nice try, though.

Foundation

I want you to throw away any painful images you have of overweight people stuffed into ill-fitting pastel leotards, sweating it out to '50s tunes under the instruction of some overcaffeinated, shorter-than-short-shorts-wearing ex-cheerleader who has more sweat bands on her body than she does muscles.

The term *aerobic* means "with oxygen," not "look like a moron." Aerobic exercise is any physical activity done for an extended period of time that forces your cardiovascular system (the heart, lungs, and blood vessels) to increase the amount of oxygen and blood circulating through your body so that you're benefitting even when you're at rest. Your body doesn't care how you make that happen, although choosing activities that work larger muscle groups, typically your legs, is more effective at getting that job done.

To count as aerobic exercise, any activity you choose has to keep your heart beating around sixty-five percent of your maximum heart rate for at least twenty minutes or more. What in Kenneth Cooper's name is your maximum heart rate? Don't worry, I'm about to explain—and it's a lot easier to follow than you think.

Your maximum heart rate, or MHR, is the highest number of times your heart can contract in one minute. To find yours, all you do is subtract your age from the number 220. That means if you're thirty-five years old, your maximum heart rate is 220 minus 35 (or

GUNNAR'S TIP

Go Long and Deep

Most people take tiny, quick steps on a stairclimber as if they're stepping on hot pavement. All those smaller steps may feel like more work, but the shorter range of motion only ends up working fewer muscle groups and burning fewer calories overall. The truth is that taking deeper steps that feel less energizing actually involves a larger percentage of muscle fibers within your gluteal muscles (butt), quadriceps, hamstrings, and calves. The more muscle fiber you can activate, the more calories your body uses for fuel.

185 beats per minute). This is an important number to know. Why? Because it can help you figure out how hard you should be exercising. To get the most from aerobic exercise, you need to keep your pulse between a range of sixty-five and eighty-five percent of that number. I recommend buying a heart rate monitor. Who are you kidding, standing on the running boards of a treadmill with your fingers pressed up against your neck while you are trying to differentiate between your pulse and the beat of the music? The monitor will make your life much easier. I also recommend figuring the sixty-five and eighty-five percent numbers that you are working to stay between and writing them on your water bottle before you get to the gym. Just a suggestion to help you focus on the task at hand.

This range (known as your *target heart rate zone*) is easier to figure out than you think. First, multiply your MHR by .65 (this number is your minimum training rate). Next, multiply your MHR again, this time by .85 (this number is your maximum training rate). The area between those two numbers is your target heart rate zone. Keep your heart rate within these numbers and you're doing enough aerobic exercise to burn fat and improve your health. Do less and you're not working hard enough to make all that effort you're putting in count the way it should.

Depending on whom you ask, most experts recommend that you need to do some form of moderate-intensity aerobic exercise at least twenty minutes a day, three days a week. Now, I'm going to be honest with you. Some people can get by on two days, so long as they never miss doing their resistance training and watch their diet. Or you may be someone who can't get the right results without putting in four days a week—or more. It depends on how committed you are to the other three wheels I'll be teaching you about later. It also depends on the type of metabolism you naturally have.

Exercising twenty minutes a day, three times a week, is a great starting point—but if you can do more, then do it. Most people approach aerobic exercise the way they leave a tip, spending the bare minimum amount of time that they can. You need to adjust this mindset. You need to look at every minute spent exercising beyond twenty minutes as another step closer to using more body fat as fuel. After that magic number (twenty minutes), you've officially exhausted your body's glycogen (carbohydrate) stores, which it uses as fuel when you work out. From a fat-burning standpoint, if you can exercise beyond twenty minutes, your body has no choice but to use more of its own stored body fat for energy instead. And you could probably tip more, too, if the service was good—but that's your call.

Need more encouragement to shoot higher than twenty? I always tell clients to pick a number between twenty-five and thirty-five that means something to them and shoot for that instead. Anything will work, from your favorite basketball or football player's jersey number to the age you wish you looked like again or the percentage you wish those shoes would go on sale. Some use their IQs, but I won't name names. Attach something personal to that higher number and you'll be more driven to reach it. It doesn't have to end in a five or a zero!

YOUR OPTIONS

Freedom

Just because whatever you're doing aerobically is working doesn't mean you shouldn't mix things up every so often. Doing the same thing day after day can make your body go postal. Instead of offing coworkers, this repeat offender–type workout takes your body hostage by figuring out an easier way to get the same job done using less effort and fewer calories. Another downside is that every activity works certain muscles and ignores others. Not switching things up can cause your body to develop imbalances.

Changing activities every few weeks can keep that from happening, but if you're really not thrilled with your options, then tweaking how you approach whatever activity you're obsessed with can help, too. Varying just one component of your aerobic exercise at a time (either the intensity, duration, or frequency) can be perceived as a change by your body without forcing you to take up an activity that you couldn't care less about.

Almost Anything Can Be Aerobic

If the whole trendy aerobics or cardio class thing isn't for you, then forget being told what to do by that microphone-wearing militia. There are hundreds of things you could do to get an aerobic workout besides using the typical gym space fillers (stationary bikes, tread-mills, stair-steppers, elliptical machines, and rowing machines) and the obvious outside choices (biking, jogging, running, swimming, and walking). All of these choices are great, but if you're not into them, that doesn't mean you should write off exercise. Playing a sport, dancing, cross-country skiing, ice-skating, kayaking, rollerblading, rock climbing, house cleaning, even gardening can all be aerobic if they are done a certain way at a certain intensity level for a certain period of time. Even the morning race to toss your disobedient kids in the car counts, as long as your heart rate was elevated throughout the whole chase!

Play to Your Strengths

Sticking to a program that you don't like may be the least effective program for you in the long run because it increases your chances of giving up on exercise altogether. Instead of picking the most popular cardio exercise now and being disappointed in your lack of attendance later, look at your body and choose exercises that will work with it instead of against it. For example, if you're too top-heavy for running, try swimming or rock climbing instead (where having a bigger upper body can be an asset). Do you have the flexibility of someone in a body cast? Then maybe skip the kickboxing at the beginning and hit the stationary cycle until you feel and move better. Have so much body fat that your nick-

GUNNAR'S TIP

Get Roped In

You don't need expensive cardio equipment to burn major calories. Skipping rope burns over 800 calories an hour, plus strengthens and works the legs from your hips to your toes. To make it easier for your body, and still burn the most calories, stick to these rules of the rope:

1. **Pick the right size.** Jump ropes may be easier to figure out compared to other machines, but you still have to adjust them to your height. Stand on the middle of the rope and raise the handles up to your chest. If they reach just below your shoulders, then it's perfect for you; if not, adjust it accordingly.

2. **No need to jump higher than one to two inches off the floor.** Not only does jumping higher place excess stress on your knees, but it actually burns fewer calories. The higher you jump, the slower you have to swing the rope around to compensate, and the fewer total jumps, which then burns fewer calories.

3. **Change your grip every few minutes.** Holding the handles so your palms face behind you, instead of in front of you, is a variation that gets some of your shoulder and back muscles into the act.

4. **Move around.** Instead of jumping straight up as the rope nears your toes, hop to your left, keeping your feet together as you go. Land on the balls of your feet, then hop back to where you were after the rope passes again. Skip normally for a few hops, then jump to the right, then back to the center again. This side-to-side variation adds an inner and outer thigh workout to the mix.

5. **Don't skip the workout just because you can't skip.** If you're not coordinated enough to skip, fake it! Just stand in place and hop up and down like you have a rope. People may think you're ready for your meds, but just mimicking the movements (minus the rope but hopping up and down at the same intensity) can still burn a good amount of calories.

name is "the before picture"? Being more buoyant can make swimming ideal for getting your heart rate up. In time, you can mix all your favorite activities and actually enjoy them, as opposed to just enduring them. I am not by any means suggesting that you bypass anything that you're not immediately suited for. I *am* saying that in the beginning, pick something that will not frustrate and annoy you so you can get into it. Then branch out. Conquer new activities as often as you can!

Pick a Low-Impact Alternative

Driving the fastest car may get you where you need to go in less time, but only if you don't blow out the engine or crash before you get there. Many high-impact exercises, such as running may burn the most calories, but they can also place a lot of stress on your joints, ligaments, tendons, and muscles. That means sticking with them may cause you to exercise less due to injury or soreness, or even worse, to quit altogether. Choosing lower-impact cardio exercises, such as step aerobics, stationary cycling, or power yoga, can also burn a large number of calories per hour. If these activities help you stay injury free and on track, you'll stay in better shape in the long run.

Be a Jet-Setter

Can't decide which type of aerobic exercise to do? Invest in a world map, tack it to a wall, and throw a dart at it. If it sticks in a water body, choose to swim or row that day. (No, that is not the universe's way of saying, "Take a relaxing bath!") If it hits on a mountain range, then switch to a stairclimber or ski machine or go on a hike. If it touches anything else, choose to cycle, walk, or run. (You could even have certain countries be certain workouts. For example, a dart in North America may mean twenty minutes of running at a high intensity, whereas a dart in South America may mean thirty minutes of running at a lower intensity. Hemispheres, baby, it's all about hemispheres!)

If you really want to set a long-term goal, find where you live on the globe and take a trip around the world, using the guidelines above. Add up the miles each week until you can officially say you've finished the ultimate race across the planet. The circumference of the earth is only 24,901 miles, so if you put in twenty miles a week, you'll hit that goal in about twenty-four years. I suggest you get going!

Use Everything in One Workout

If you want a workout your body will never get used to (or forgive you for), try flip-flopping between your cardio choices at the gym (stationary bike, treadmill, step routine, jump rope, stairclimber) every three minutes. Make the first minute a warm-up, push yourself around sixty-five percent of your MHR for the second minute, then go all out if you're up for it (eighty to eighty-five percent of your MHR) for the last minute.

Move Things Around

If you typically use the Lifecycle that's third from the right at your gym, try the one next to it and keep working your way down the line every few days. If you exercise at home, turn your cardiovascular machine to face another direction or move it altogether. A new view, even one that's off by a few degrees in any direction, can make each experience feel different enough to alleviate boredom and keep you exercising longer.

Focus

Monitoring your heart rate may already feel fairly high maintenance, and you might feel like it requires enough focus on your part. But if you can eke out a bit more concentration to play with your heart rate every once in a while, you may find yourself burning even more calories in the long run.

Go Slowly Once in a While

Occasionally picking a new activity that only raises your heart rate between fifty and sixty percent of your MHR may seem less effective, but it's also a pace that's easier to maintain for a longer period of time. With most aerobic exercises, you may actually burn more calories at this pace, if you take advantage of the slower tempo and double your workout time. For example, sprint at eight mph (a 7.5-minute-mile pace) and you may burn 300 calories in thirty minutes, but you'll probably pass out directly afterward. Compare that with jogging slowly (at five mph) and you'll not only last an hour, but also burn over 350 calories instead.

GUNNAR'S TIP

Turn Your Workout Around

Try standing on your stairclimber or treadmill facing the opposite direction. The move may feel awkward and you may look stupid, but this position strengthens the legs from a different angle that places more emphasis on the front of your legs (quadriceps) rather than on the back of them (glutes and hamstrings). This can be done at intervals during your regular workouts or for the entire workout from time to time.

Go Fast Once in a While

The flip side of going slow once in a while to mix things up is occasionally going faster than usual to give your body a change. If you're healthy enough to do it, you can actually burn *more* overall calories when you exercise over seventy-five percent of your MHR. Not only will you burn more calories by maintaining a higher intensity, but pushing yourself at this level causes your body to reach for calories from stored carbohydrates— which are easier for your body to process for instant energy—instead of using stored body fat. That may sound counterproductive, but it still leads to fat loss, since the fewer excess calories you have in your body after your workout, the less your body has to convert into body fat later on.

Building up to that type of intensity isn't something you should try too quickly. To get your body used to working at that pace, try exercising at sixty-five percent for two minutes, then raise the intensity up to seventy-five percent for thirty seconds, then lower the intensity back down to sixty-five percent. Keep flip-flopping between sixty-five percent and seventy-five percent for the length of your twenty-minute workout. As you get in better shape, start shortening the time you work at sixty-five percent a few seconds each workout. Once you can exercise regularly for a total of thirty minutes—alternating between one minute at sixty-five percent and thirty seconds at seventy-five percent of your MHR—your body should be ready to handle a twenty-minute workout at seventy-five percent intensity.

Know When Too Much Is Too Much

Pushing yourself higher within your target heart rate zone will definitely reap more results, but you need to know when too much is too much. If you can't speak a full sentence while exercising without being winded, like "Call 9–1–1, please . . . ," you're most likely pushing yourself toward the far end of your target heart rate zone. On the other hand, if you're able to carry on a full conversation with someone about the amazing acting range of Scooby

GUNNAR'S TIP

Tilt Your Treadmill

Whenever you walk (or run) outside, you're pulling yourself forward. But because a treadmill's motor pulls the surface along, it prevents your legs from working as hard as they should, so it's almost as if you're walking on a slight downgrade. Raising the treadmill to a one percent incline can prevent that downhill force against the knee, helping you overcome your own body weight against gravity so your muscles work just as hard as they would on a flat surface outside.

Doo, you're probably working at a level that's below your target heart rate zone (not to mention, you're probably not a very good judge of talent, but that's nothing I can help you with).

FREQUENTLY ASKED QUESTIONS

1. "Can I be too old for aerobic exercise?"

There are things that old(er) people would be well advised to avoid—streaking across football fields and wearing short-shorts come to mind—but aerobic exercise isn't on the list. There's a good chance that one of the reasons you *feel* old is because you're *not* doing any form of cardiovascular training in the first place. In fact, aerobic exercise has been shown to be beneficial for people suffering from a variety of medical disorders such as heart disease, diabetes, obesity, arthritis, and anxiety. It does nothing for baldness, though. Sorry.

Still, if you're over forty or have a known history of heart disease, high blood pressure, or any other cardiovascular disorder, check in with whichever white coat takes a look at you from time to time and see what he or she thinks first. A doctor can help determine the best answer for you based on a few key factors, such as your age, sex, weight, diet, and lifestyle.

2. "Is walking really considered aerobic exercise?"

The mention of walking as a means of exercise may conjure images of obsessed blue-haired power walkers, marching through malls like some sort of senior-citizen brigade. For some intermediate exercisers, the main misconception about walking is that it's just too effortless to be considered exercise.

Sure, it's one of the lowest-ranking cardio exercises when it comes to burning calories (200 to 300 an hour—a ballpark figure), but on the flip side, it also poses the least amount of health risks of almost any cardiovascular activity. Besides, your heart isn't keeping score of what you're doing to work it either. It could care less whether you're running a marathon or walking up a large hill, barring the deleterious effects on your joints. All it knows is that you're raising your heart rate and maintaining it at that level for at least twenty minutes. You'll improve your cardiovascular abilities significantly, even if the race is over, everyone's gone, and you're the last one across the finish line. By the way, who cares?

3. "If I can't exercise for at least twenty minutes, is it a waste of my time?"

First of all, if you really can't find twenty minutes, three times a week, the first thing we need to discuss is your time management skills and your priorities. With our crazy schedules these days, having time requires making time: It's as simple as that. Sure, that might mean pulling yourself out of bed as soon as the alarm goes off (rather than hitting snooze five times) and devoting the early morning to your workout. It might mean flipping off the sitcoms in the evening and using that time to get your heart rate up. You know your schedule best. But don't give me the "not enough time" cop out—you make time for so many other things in your day, why not give priority to your body and your health? And if you're still not sure you can squeeze it in, think of it this way: Adding in exercise will improve your focus, heighten your productivity, and improve your energy—in short, the time spent will more than make up for itself during the rest of your day.

That said, I know there are those days—and from time to time, those weeks—when you really *can't* find the time to stick to your plans. Just because you may not have enough time to exercise for twenty minutes doesn't mean it's not worth breaking a sweat at all! Having only ten minutes to spend on aerobic training is still like working a half day. You may not be making as much money that day, but c'mon, you're still getting paid! And you feel better for having done something, not to mention for being seen at the office!

It's true that your body burns a greater percentage of body fat when you exercise for twenty minutes and beyond (instead of glycogen, your body burns carbohydrates that it stores to use for short-term energy). But you still burn the same amount of calories by dividing your workout into shorter periods of time (even if that's two ten-minute sessions, four five-minute workouts, or even ten two-minute bursts). In fact, since your metabolism temporarily revs up after you exercise, studies have shown that dividing your workouts may even burn more total calories. By breaking things up, you're able to speed up your metabolism more than once a day for more results, even if you're using less fat for energy.

GUNNAR'S TIP

Confuse Your Feet

If you feel your walks are getting a bit lame, try moving them to an unstable terrain instead. Soft sand, waist-high water, tall grass, steep hills, narrow curbs, and loose rocks are just a few of the ways to change the intensity of an otherwise dull workout. With every shaky step, your body has to activate more proprioceptive muscles (the mini-stabilizers that maintain balance and muscular control) throughout your entire body just to keep itself stable. Constantly working these balance adjusters not only burns a few extra calories, but it teaches your body to recover during other activities or sports that may challenge your balance.

Of all the cardio exercises out there, running is considered by many to be the end-all-be-all if the goal is to drop pounds fast. There's no denying that running burns an average of 600 to 800 calories an hour, but so do other high-impact exercises (including skipping rope and intense step classes). You can even get the same calorie-burning benefits of high-impact exercise in a low-impact activity, such as cross-country skiing or swimming. Both activities burn plenty of calories by working the upper and lower body simultaneously (running predominantly works your lower body) without placing your joints or spine under any unnecessary stress.

I'm not trying to discourage anyone from running, but it's far from the only option. The truth is that any activity that causes your heart and lungs to work harder to provide more oxygen to your muscles for an extended period of time could be aerobic enough to be more effective than running. So whether you simply hate the thought of logging miles or you have bad knees or other problems that prevent you from getting mileage, don't despair: Running is just one of many things a person can do to lose weight.

The Second Wheel: Resistance Training

Resistance training.

Whether you're brand new to this whole exercise experience or fitness is old hat, you probably still know what resistance training entails, or know it by one of its many other names: strength training, weight training, pumping iron, anaerobic exercise.

Do any of these ring a bell?

This is the chapter you've either been waiting for or dreading since the very first page. If you're male and breathing, you may start to get a bit fired up now. If you're female, and fairly new to fitness, you might have doubts, or even visions of morphing into a 300-pound monster with arms like hamhocks as soon as you start bench pressing. Relax, it's not like that.

THE FACTS

Function

Resistance training is not just about building muscle that will help you look great. It's also what I call "pre-hab" for preventing injuries and making sure you feel great. Research has shown that strength training at least three times a week can reduce levels of LDL cholesterol (the bad, artery-clogging kind) and help reduce your risk of developing a number of health conditions, including diabetes, cardiovascular disease, osteoporosis, and some forms of cancer. Resistance training also turns back the clock by reversing many factors that naturally occur in the aging process. Decreased mobility, loss of balance, joint instability, and loss of muscle tissue are just a handful of aging side effects that lifting a little weight on a regular basis can actually reverse, no matter when you start. (It has even resulted in improvements in 100-year-olds!)

Would you rather do resistance training *now* to stave off health risks or have some uptight physician prescribe it to you as "rehab" therapy when you're walking around hunched over from bad health habits later on? I don't know about you, but avoiding an injury is always preferable to me to dealing with injury, not to mention it saves a visit to the doctor and the ensuing lecture.

Reshaping your muscles can even help you stay leaner. Aerobic exercise burns more calories per minute and gets your metabolism into overdrive faster than resistance training, which burns fewer calories and raises your metabolism only slightly. However, after you've done your weight training, your body has to use extra calories throughout the day just to sustain the new, leaner body you've built for yourself. Using weights effectively will keep your metabolism turned on all day long.

So think of muscle as the fat-burning friend who's with you all day long. The more muscle you have, the higher your basal metabolic rate (BMR). What's a BMR, and why should you care about it? Your BMR is another important number: It is the number of calories you burn every day just to keep your body functioning, your heart beating, your lungs breathing, and so on. It's your BMR that accounts for almost seventy-five percent of all of the calories you burn daily, with the other twenty-five percent being burned from all your daily physical activities.

Building more muscle through resistance training means you'll have extra muscle fibers consuming more energy, even when they're just sitting there looking good but not doing a damn thing. In fact, every pound of muscle you add to your frame burns an additional thirty to fifty calories per day. Substitute five pounds of muscle on your frame for five pounds of sagging fat and not only will you naturally be more aesthetically in shape, but you'll burn an extra 150 to 250 calories a day doing absolutely nothing at all. It's your fat-burning sidekick, doing all the dirty work for you long after you stop exercising.

Foundation

No matter what name you use, resistance training is a form of anaerobic exercise. What's the difference between aerobic and anaerobic exercise besides a couple of extra letters at the front of the word? You already know that aerobic exercise is any activity that increases your pulse for an extended period of time, causing your heart and lungs to work harder to get more oxygen to your muscles. Well, anaerobic exercise is any activity done in short, intense bursts that works your body *without* requiring much oxygen.

That's what you're doing whenever you lift weights, pull on stretch cords, or do anything in an attempt to shape your muscles. Resistance training means working one muscle (or a group of muscles) against some form of resistance so that your muscles have no choice but to break down from fatigue and stress. Do it the right way, and those beaten-down muscles of yours have no choice but to rebuild themselves so they're stronger for the next time you decide to put them through the paces.

It doesn't matter what form of resistance you use to get the job done. Your muscles don't care if the weight you're lifting has been rusting away in your basement for decades or if it's one of those nice, available-in-ten-pastel-colors dumbbell sets intended to make you forget that they're weights. No matter what tool you use to stress your muscles—barbells, dumbbells, weight machines, stretch cords, medicine balls, your own body weight—if you provide enough resistance to fatigue your muscles by making them repeat a movement for a given number of repetitions, you'll achieve the same goal.

Here's how it works: Lifting the weight one time is called a **repetition**. A group of repetitions performed without stopping is called a **set**. The number of repetitions you should do to fatigue your muscles depends on your goals. Most experts stick with using a weight you can lift, raise, or pull eight to fifteen times. If you're looking to noticeably strengthen your muscles, then using a heavier weight that allows you to do only between six and ten repetitions is better. If improving muscular endurance is your goal—meaning, you want muscles that won't tire out when you're playing sports or being active—plan on beginning with your body weight, then progressing to a lighter weight that lets you do twelve to twenty or more repetitions.

Before any resistance training workout, you need to do some form of mild aerobic exercise to help warm up your muscles. Just doing five minutes of a low-intensity cardiovascular exercise (cycling in low gear, walking in place, or pretending you know how to jump rope) is fine. What this does is raise the temperature of your muscles, which can decrease your risk of injury by making them more pliable. This extra flexibility provides muscles with a greater range of motion, letting you activate more muscle fibers as you exercise.

YOUR OPTIONS

Freedom

The choices you have with resistance training are virtually limitless—so much so that I had to give them their own chapter. Soon, I'll be showing you how to create hundreds and hundreds of exercises that will prevent your muscles from ever being bored again. But for now, just know that I won't be disappointing you.

Resistance training isn't just about putting in the numbers. Does the slacker who shows up to work just so he can be seen from nine to five get the same bonuses, raises, and company perks as the guy who shows up from nine to five and makes every hour count? It's not just about the numbers; it's about making every number count. Exercise imitates life.

If resistance training's never worked for you and you use perfect form (something I'll show you later in this book), I would bet my dog that you're using weights that are too light for you. It's the mistake I try to never let happen in my gym. But if you don't have someone bulldogging you, it's a lot easier for your muscles to skate by. Guess what—I'm not going to let that happen here either.

If you're not using a weight heavy enough to fully fatigue your muscles during each set, you'll never push them enough to make them want, and need, to improve themselves. For example, if an exercise asks you to do twelve to fifteen repetitions, you need to select a weight that you can complete only twelve to fifteen repetitions with while still keeping good form. If you could have easily eked out three more repetitions beyond that before quitting, your muscles were never really challenged enough to improve themselves, making the entire set less effective than it should and certainly could have been. Once you can do more than the required number of repetitions, then it's time to raise the weight you're using by one to five pounds or increase the number of reps (depending on the exercise and the targeted muscle group). You will still get something out of the work even if you are not reaching failure, but when you push it you will get so much more.

FREQUENTLY ASKED QUESTIONS

1. "Won't weights make me big?"

If you're a guy, you can probably skip over this question. Go on—see you in a minute. If you're a woman, do me a favor and read up on me to see all the women I've worked with over the years. See anyone who ever looked like a linebacker in a dress? No one, right? I didn't think so. And every single woman who works with me has no choice but to hit the weights to some degree every time she comes into my gym. Look, I know, I know, I know. You don't want to get heavy. You don't want to be bulky. You don't want to be a big, muscular mess! I've got a news flash coming straight off the wire that's meant just for you:

YOU WON'T!!!

I can promise you that I could have you lift everything in this world that's heavy as many times as you can heave it and you will not get huge. As a rule, that's because most women are simply not genetically capable of ballooning up from strength training alone.

Your body has around ten percent of the testosterone that the average male has—and just look at how those knuckleheads struggle to put on extreme muscle. Even *they* can't do it, and they're trying every day! So what do you think your chances are of getting that big?

Just because you saw someone who was huge doing an exercise you were thinking of trying doesn't mean you're going to look like that person after doing that same exercise. That same approach doesn't work for aerobic exercise, does it? *No* is the answer in case you were struggling. You can't jump on the same bike that some svelte, tight-bodied model just rode for sixty minutes and expect to look like her just because you're using something she uses! It doesn't work for hairbrushes or toothpaste either. Please don't shoot the messenger.

The truth is, even if you work your muscles to extreme fatigue, the vast majority of women are genetically incapable of creating large, bulky muscles, because they lack sufficient hormones or even the body structure to support that type of muscle tissue. Unless you are chemically enhancing your testosterone levels, resistance training (no matter what you choose to lift) will only create stronger, denser, shapelier muscles.

Oh, and if you're worried that adding a pound of muscle is still a pound, it's estimated that the "space" of a pound of muscle is about twenty-two percent less than a pound of fat. That means adding five pounds of muscle and losing five pounds of fat would actually make you look smaller. I'd say that's a fair trade-off.

Finally, muscle is not created by weights. It's created by food—proteins, to be more precise. You have to eat a quality and quantity of food above and beyond what you burn, plus break the muscles down in the gym so that they need to repair, plus eat every three to four hours, plus get adequate rest so that they can recover, plus . . . do you see what I mean? Besides, if it started to happen, it's not an overnight process, so you could always back off or even stop. More on this later, but for now, just trust me.

2. "Can I burn fat from a specific area by doing specific exercises?"

Welcome to the biggest con in fitness and exercise. It may be the quick fix you're wishing for, but spot reduction (the popular term for it) is one of the biggest exercise lies out there.

It's impossible to lose weight in one particular area by lifting weights or doing exercises that target only that area. Your body burns all its fat in a genetically predetermined pattern over which you have no control. But there's good news: As you start driving on all four wheels, you'll begin to burn fat gradually from all over your body, including your specific wish list of areas.

Typically, the last place you store fat is the first area you'll see a noticeable difference. If that was the fourth chin you developed last week, chances are that chin will quickly be returned to its rightful pelican once you take action. Unfortunately, that also means the first place you started storing fat is usually the last area to get lean. If you're a man, that's typically right around your waist; if you're a woman, then we're probably talking about that butt or those hips.

Are all those exercises that claim to "spot reduce" fat useless? Not all of them, if you're legitimately feeling the muscles working and contracting when you're doing them. But what you're doing is improving the shape and density of those muscles beneath the blubber, or subcutaneous fat. Until you reduce the body fat above or around your muscles—through cardiovascular exercise, resistance training, eating right, and adequate rest—you'll never make them more pronounced and visible. You may naturally *have* a perfect set of abs under your belly and not even know it because you like to double down on your take-out. If you want to find out for yourself, it's still not going to happen unless you're willing to drive on all four wheels and stop putting blind faith in what others are trying to sell you.

3. "I just want to sculpt and tone my muscles. How do I do that?"

Hot button! I'm about to burst your bubble again on many levels. Sculpt, tone, lengthen, and every other sexy expression you've ever heard used to describe building muscle are pure spin. Here's why you can't believe everything you read.

You can't lengthen a muscle!

Ever see an ad for a machine or read about an exercise or a workout "system" that offers you long, lean muscles? Then you're reading something written by someone either clueless about anatomy or trying to sell you a promise he or she can't possibly keep.

The truth is that the length of each and every muscle within your body is purely genetic. You are born with origins of muscles and insertions of muscles where the muscles you have connect to the bones you have. That's it. That means the only shot you ever had at lengthening your muscles was way back when your parents were working up a sweat on their own.

Most exercise bullshit artists and snake oil salespeople will claim that certain exercises that work your muscles through a full range of motion can lengthen them. Although getting yourself in certain positions (which I'll show you later in this book) can make it easier to work a muscle more thoroughly, nothing short of my chaining you to some medieval torture rack will *ever* lengthen your muscles. Period. End of story.

You can't tone or sculpt a muscle!

Yeah, yeah, yeah. I know you've read about it a million times. Using the right exercises can sculpt your problem areas and tone your muscles. But let's get one thing straight: Your body isn't a sculpture slapped together with clay, ready to be cut, carved, and chiseled. It's not a sack of stuff that a few exercises can easily shift around. Your body, minus about 206 bones and a few major organs, is basically skin, fat, and muscle. It's how much you have of the last two that has *anything* to do with how your muscles appear from the outside.

All those words are just pathetic euphemisms to appease those who really don't want to commit to exercise. Sexy muscles! Toned muscles! Sculpted muscles! Lean muscles! Shapely muscles! For some reason, someone decided that you'd want to hear softer words that sound less difficult or threatening, and more appealing, and ever since then they've all pitched it that way. The truth is, whenever anyone refers to toned, sexy, sculpted, lean (that one's funny—muscle *is* lean by its very nature), or shapely muscle, they're talking about giving your muscles a contracted, visible appearance. From a visual perspective, what they're promising are muscles with more shape and contour. Well, the only way to see those muscles is to get rid of excess body fat through better nutrition and exercise. And the only way to guarantee your muscles will have a desirable shape (by this I mean size and proportion vis-à-vis the rest of your body, other muscles included) when the fat disappears is through resistance training. That's reality talking, not some cover line written to sell magazines or supplements.

The next time you see an exercise regimen that promises to "tone" or "sculpt" your muscles, take a closer look to see if they bother to mention anything about aerobic exercise or how to eat healthy. Chances are that advice is never mentioned, or is cleverly tucked away in a one-line disclaimer.

Throughout this book, you'll never see any of the words I've just mentioned unless I'm ripping on them with good reason. I don't use them with my athletes and actors, and their bodies are living proof that hearing the real facts about exercise is what truly pays off. If you're going to take resistance training seriously, just remember: If you want soft words, you'll have a soft body. If you're ready to accept the hard truth, then you're ready to develop a hard body.

4. "Can I really get results without going to a gym?"

My facility is packed with top-of-the-line equipment, but you don't need a big, full gym to stay in shape. Eleven of the thirteen basic exercises I'm about to show you can be done with just a set of dumbbells, a flat bench, and an exercise mat. The other two can be done with a simple high-cable accessory that attaches at the end of an adjustable bench, or you can use resistance bands. Obviously, my vote is for you to get to the gym. It's just better. I know the saying "More is not always better," but when it comes to exercise equipment, yes it is, in my opinion, because it gives you choices and helps stave off boredom! But you can and must get it done even if it has to be at home. Period.

5. "Is this going to hurt my back?"

If I had a dollar for every time I heard this, John Kerry would have proposed to me.

Let me tell you my own little "back story" first. The pain was intermittent at first, and I assumed it was nothing. Then it became constant and I thought maybe it was the leg presses I was doing. Turns out it wasn't. I varied my training program. I even took a couple of days off. I tried pushing through it. I tried working around it. I got a new mattress. I walked into a "Relax the Back" store set on solving this problem and spent $850 on different items from pillows to massagers. I tried chiropractic visits, traction, acupuncture, magnetic therapy, inversion boots, and just plain old massage. Then I started going to doctors. I saw three orthopedic surgeons who told me that I needed an operation because I had a disk bulge (also called protrusion or herniation). I even got three separate epidural cortisone shots. Those were fun. Each worked to a varying degree for a period of time, but eventually they all wore off.

Then I saw a neurosurgeon who said that I had a broken vertebra that had slipped forward and "fallen off." That had to hurt. I had broken my wrists three times, my ribs twice, and my nose, but this was new and I didn't remember an incident when it happened. You would think I would remember that, wouldn't you? He said it happens over time and that it was not due to something I did. Whew! Now I felt better. But my back still hurt—a lot. He said that while I did have a disk bulge, that was a red herring and only part of what was going on back there. He said that I needed an operation or I would lose control of my bowels. Well, actually, he said that I needed an operation or I would develop more of a foot drop, which I would compensate for with my gait, which would cause other biomechanical problems. Then I would probably develop a foot drop on the other side, then lose bladder control, and eventually lose control of my bowels. There's a bad look for your trainer, huh?

I got one more opinion from another neurosurgeon who said that the first neurosurgeon was right and that he was a great doctor and a pioneer in his field. I went back to him and asked about what I would lose in terms of ability and mobility if I went through with the surgery. He said that I would have 100 percent recovery. I asked for his definition of 100 percent, because some of the other doctors had me playing shuffleboard and training in a pool for the rest of my life. He said, "You can ski the bumps and practice full-contact martial arts, if you want." "I want," I said. He explained that recovery time varied but that I could expect to be out of the hospital in a week and back in the gym in six months. That was hard to swallow, but he was wearing the lab coat, so who was I to argue? I had been in constant pain for eighteen months at this point. I couldn't stand upright without holding on to something. I had to lean all the time. Great look for someone in fitness. I knew I had to have the surgery when I was holding my eight-month-old baby boy and I had to kneel down after fifteen seconds because the pain was so excruciating. By the way, I was still training eight to ten people a day through this pain. My spotting techniques may have looked strange, but I was never unsafe. I leaned on equipment, knelt down, and braced myself between barbell racks—whatever it took so that no one would know about the pain. The trainer can't be hurt!

The surgery lasted six hours and involved opening me up in back, pulling the "fallen" vertebra up, using a titanium plate with four screws to hold it in place, drilling a hole on each side in the foramen, then flipping me over, opening me up, putting a cage in the gap under the vertebra that was pulled back, packing it with cadaver marrow (nice), and putting one last screw in to hold the cage in place. The pain was the worst for first twenty-four hours post-op, and I thought I was going to die from it. I am such a baby. I decided that the hospital was not the place for me, but the doctor wouldn't sign off on my release until I could walk around the hall (God, that hall seemed long!) without my walker. My walker—another good look for a trainer. I made that my goal, and I pushed. Laps became reps; the walker became my training partner—a training partner I soon outgrew. I was out of the hospital in four days and riding a stationary bike in ten days. I was lifting weights in twelve days. He was shocked, amazed, wary, and impressed. He became my friend and my client, and he even did a testimonial in my Core Secrets™ infomercial! His name is Dr. Robert Bray, and, as far as I am concerned, you can call him God. He saved my life in a number of ways. I have no physical restrictions other than being a terrible basketball player, but I make up for that with energy and passion. And I now have empirical data about what the human body can do, go through, and recover from. My first pain-free day felt like I had rented someone else's body. The sensation was as foreign as the downtime post-op had been. I could not believe it. I was back, and, in fact, I was better than ever. All thanks to Dr. Robert Bray.

Now, tell me about your back pain. I think we can find a way to make it better. . . .

THE LUCKY THIRTEEN

You can't move ahead until you take the first step forward.

Children learn to crawl before they learn to walk. Runners take up jogging before they run races. Politicians learn to run races before they apologize on national television for lying and other scandalous acts.

When it comes to entering the intimidating world of resistance training, the same rules apply. Before you venture off into trying fitness moves that look more like a contortionist's warm-up than exercise, the smartest thing you can do is master the basic movements first. In fact, it's the only move you can make if you're in this long term. Abandoning the basics makes it too easy to stray from achieving a total body balance, since most people tend to tailor their workouts around whichever body part they think needs the most improvement. However, there's another very important reason to focus on the basics.

Here's what way too many personal trainers don't want you to know. About eighty-five to ninety percent of any flashy exercise you see hyped as the "new way to get in shape" is a spin-off of a classic move you must know how to do properly first.

That's right.

Thousands of those newfound miracle moves you've read about that promise to tone up your abs, work off your butt, and supposedly "sculpt" (I really, really don't like that word!) your arms are really just spin-offs from thirteen main exercises. Don't get me wrong, all these "spin-offs" have their place down the road. But by learning these Lucky Thirteen moves first, you can cut through the confusion about which exercise spin-offs are right for you. You will finally get it, and you'll get more out of the spin-off when you are really ready to try it.

Understanding how to do the Lucky Thirteen with perfect form will not only get you started on the path to the body you want, but it'll also give you the power to create thousands of exercise options later on. Basically, it's *my* guarantee that you'll never stop seeing results. How can I promise that? Easy. Because you'll never have the same workout twice. I don't, my clients don't, so why should you?

If you're green to weight lifting, these Lucky Thirteen exercises are all you'll need to get started. If you're an advanced exerciser, you're about to rethink everything you thought you knew about exercise, and you'll love doing it.

Getting Started

The best resistance-training workout leaves no stone unturned. It's a program that targets every major muscle group in your body, not just the ones you're concerned with. The Lucky Thirteen are the best overall muscle-developing exercises with the most versatility. They're the force behind G-Force.

> For your legs and butt: The squat and the lunge
>
> For your chest: The chest press and the chest fly
>
> For your back: The pulldown and the row
>
> For your shoulders: The shoulder press and the raise
>
> For your triceps: The pressdown and the extension
>
> For your biceps: The curl
>
> For your abs: The crunch and the reverse crunch

Are there any exercises I've left out? If you're not that new to exercise, I'm sure you'll find a few right off the bat. Here, I'll give you a couple right now before you discover them yourself, just so you don't think I slipped. You won't find the leg extension, the leg curl, the upright row, the hyperextension, the shrug, and a few others. But let me ask you this: Would you rather learn one exercise that can teach you only a handful of new spin-offs that you may be able to do only in a gym, or would you rather learn one exercise that gives you hundreds of spin-offs that you can do anywhere?

I'll wait right here until you make up your mind.

Welcome back. That was fast.

Now, let's get started on learning how to do the Lucky Thirteen with the same perfect form I expect from every actor, actress, athlete, businesswoman, stay-at-home dad, trusta-farian, doctor, lawyer, singer, accountant, consultant, and even personal trainer that I have been lucky enough to have worked with over the years.

Before You Begin, You Better Be Doing This . . .

One of the essential steps toward getting in shape is avoiding injury. The smartest thing you can do with any exercise is to listen to your body. If something hurts or doesn't feel right, your body's probably trying to tell you you're doing something wrong. When you begin exercising, pay attention to your pain. Experiencing muscle soreness during or following a workout is perfectly normal. That's because contracting a muscle past its threshold causes waste material and other acids to build up inside of it.

Experiencing this burning sensation means your muscles are getting their money's worth. However, if you feel a muscle start to cramp, stop what you're doing, drink some water, and gently move the muscle until it unwinds itself. If you feel any sharp, continuous pain during any exercise or a pain that persists after a few days, stop your resistance training immediately and have yourself checked out by a doctor (just to be on the safe side).

There are a few common rules that must be followed strictly no matter what exercise you use to work your muscles. Read this list carefully and you'll be much better off in the long run.

Your head: Unless I say otherwise, your head should always face forward and be kept in a direct line with your spine. Turning your head to the left, right, up, or down will only place unnecessary stress on your joints and neck muscles, which are usually contracting during most exercises. I should always be able to place a tennis ball right under your chin.

Your back: Unless I tell you to flex or extend your spine, your back should be kept in a straight line throughout any exercise. Picture a bar running from the top of your head straight down to your coccyx (tailbone). Arching your back or rolling it forward only makes it easier to use momentum to rob you from seeing results, plus it can increase your risk of injury.

Your wrists: Keep your wrists in line with your forearms at all times. Bending them forward or backward as you raise, pull, or push a weight will only redirect pressure onto the weaker tendons and muscles within your wrists and forearms.

Your hands: Grab a weight only as tightly as you need to so that you don't drop it. Gripping too tightly only makes the tiny muscles within your wrists, hands, and forearms work constantly. This is usually a co-contraction, which is your body's response to or anticipation of stress. Keeping that death grip going throughout every exercise will only cause those smaller muscles to peter out before the bigger muscles you're trying to work ever get a chance to do their thing.

Your elbows and knees: Whenever any exercise asks you to straighten your arms or legs, you don't need to extend them so far that your elbows or knees lock out. Doing this takes the effort of any exercise away from the muscles you're trying to work and places more of it on your joints, which are not as strong.

Your feet: Unless you're being asked to raise your feet or stand on one of them, both of your feet should be pressed flat on the floor at all times. Shifting around, raising up on your toes, or rearing back on your heels is generally a sign that you're trying to cheat by positioning other muscles to help out (the exception, of course, being when a move requires an unusual foot position, such as a lunge or twisting movement).

THE MOVES

1. THE SQUAT

What It's Working

The quadriceps, gluteal muscles, and calves, as well as the core muscles—the ones tucked along your spine and wrapped around your torso, including your lower back, and abdominals—that are responsible for stabilizing your midsection.

Do the Move

Stand with your feet shoulder-width apart and a barbell resting across the back of your shoulders. (If you have a squat rack, grab the bar with an overhand grip slightly wider than shoulder-width apart, duck underneath it, and rest the bar across the back of your shoulders.) With your back straight and feet shoulder-width apart, slowly squat down until your thighs are almost parallel to the floor. Slowly push yourself back up into a standing position and repeat.

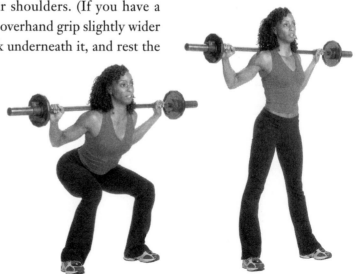

Feel the Move

As you squat down, imagine that you're about to sit in a chair, keeping your back straight, eyes straight ahead, and your body weight spread from your heels to the balls of your feet. As you push yourself back up, imagine you have a rope around your belt buckle and someone's tugging on it from the ceiling to pull you up. Think about actively pushing through your heels.

The Mistakes Everybody Makes

Don't snap into a locked-out knee position at the top. Locking the knees takes the load of the weight off your glutes, hamstrings, and quadriceps and redirects that pressure onto your knees and lower back. Making them as straight as you can *without* locking your knees keeps your muscles contracted, forcing them to work even harder so you don't have to spend as much time trying to exhaust them.

Don't lean forward. If you have a logo on your shirt or if you are wearing a necklace, you should be able to see it in the mirror during the movement. Nothing like a little "bling" on your leg day! If you can't see it in the mirror as you squat, that means you're either leaning too far forward or you've dropped your head down.

Keep your feet facing forward, but stick with what's comfortable for you. Imagine you're standing on a big clock with the 12 right in front of you. Pointing your left foot between 11 and 12 and your right foot between 12 and 1 is perfectly fine if you have a hard time pointing both feet straight ahead.

If you feel all your weight on the balls of your feet, you're leaning too far forward and not letting your butt sink down properly. Think about trying to press your heels into the floor as if you were going to jump up but changed your mind at the last minute. Use your power!

2. THE LUNGE

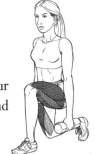

What It's Working

Glutes (the muscles that make up your butt), hamstrings (your back thigh muscles), quadriceps (your front thigh muscles), and calves (the lower leg muscles).

Do the Move

Stand with a dumbbell in each hand, arms hanging at your sides and your feet about hip-width apart. Keeping your back straight, take a normal step backward with your left foot. When the ball of your left foot touches the floor, continue the movement by lowering your hips until your right thigh becomes parallel to the floor. Your right knee should be bent at almost a ninety-degree angle with your right knee directly above your right foot. Gently push yourself back into the starting position by driving the right foot into the floor and repeat the move, this time stepping back with your right foot. Continue the exercise by alternating between your left and right leg.

Feel the Move

To really feel this exercise, don't concentrate on the leg that's behind you; focus on the leg that's in front of you. Even though it stays in place, it's actually the one that's working as you lower yourself down. I want you to push that forward foot through the floor to make you stand and to bring you back to the starting position.

The Mistakes Everyone Makes

Don't lean too far forward. Your weight needs to stay on your heels. Shifting too far forward transfers your weight onto your toes, putting excessive torque on your knee joint. Instead, always keep your knee directly over your toes. One way to spot-check yourself: Perform the exercise standing sideways to a mirror so you can watch how far you come down.

3. THE CHEST PRESS

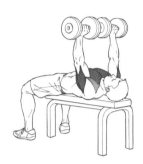

What It's Working

Pectoralis major and pectoralis minor (chest), the front head of your shoulders, and the triceps (the muscles in the back of your arms).

Do the Move

Lie face up on a flat exercise bench (shown below on stability ball) with your knees bent and feet flat on the floor. Grab a dumbbell in each hand and position them along the sides of your chest, palms facing forward. Your elbows should be pointing toward the floor. This is the starting position of the move. Now, slowly press the weights straight up until your arms are fully extended above your chest, elbows barely unlocked. Squeeze your chest muscles for a second, then slowly lower the dumbbells back along the sides of your chest.

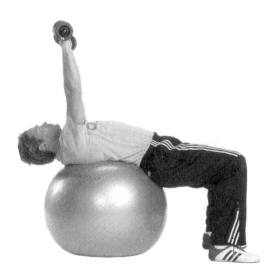

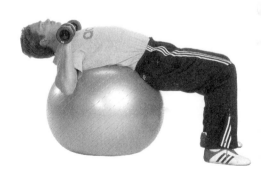

Feel the Move

At the top of the movement, I tell my clients to squeeze their chest muscles as though they were trying to create cleavage. C'mon, you know that's why you're doing it in the first place! Still, this tip does more than help you focus on the muscles you're working; it actually forces more muscle fibers in your chest to contract, which can yield better results.

The Mistakes Everybody Makes

Keep your back and head flat on the bench throughout the exercise, but don't worry too much if your back doesn't feel completely flattened on the bench. We all have a natural curve to our spines, so trying to press yourself too hard against the bench will only compromise your form. Just try to avoid arching your back (which helps other muscles cheat the weight up), and you'll be fine.

Don't bring the weights down farther than the outer edges of your chest. By lowering the weights below your chest, your arms have no choice but to bend at an angle less than ninety degrees. Once your arms bend at an angle of ninety degrees or less, your chest muscles lose their ability to contract properly, causing the effort of supporting the weight to shift to smaller, weaker muscles within the shoulder joint.

Never let the elbows get in front of or in back of your wrists. By letting your elbows shift in either direction, you place your body at a mechanical disadvantage and shift the stress to your shoulder muscles. Your forearms should stay perpendicular to the floor.

Control the weight on the way down. If you're using a barbell or heavier weights, or just have a large chest so that the weights (or bar) have no choice but to touch your chest on the lowering phase, make sure the weight doesn't slam into your body. Just let it lightly touch your chest before pressing the weight back up.

4. THE CHEST FLY

What It's Working

Pectoralis major and pectoralis minor (chest), the front head of the shoulders, and the serratus anterior muscles (the muscles along your rib cage).

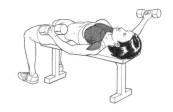

Do the Move

Grab a pair of light dumbbells and lie on your back on a flat exercise bench. Extend your arms straight up above your chest. The weights should be together with your palms facing each other, elbows unlocked. This is the starting position of the move. Now, slowly lower the dumbbells out to your sides in a semicircular arc until they're as low as comfortably possible. Slowly bring your arms back up (again, in an arclike sweep) until the weights are once again above your chest. Repeat.

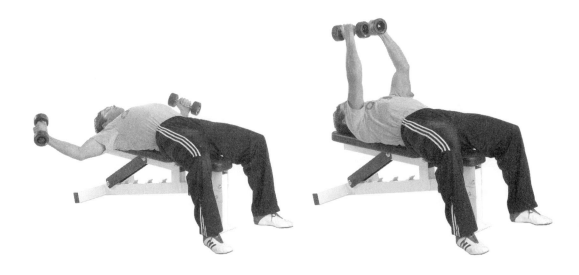

Feel the Move

As you sweep your arms out to the sides, picture yourself hugging a large tree. That's how wide you want to keep your arms as you lower the weights. Once the weights meet at the top, try creating cleavage again like you did for the chest press.

The Mistakes Everybody Makes

Be sure not to lock your elbows during the movement; that will take the tension off the pectorals and deliver it to your joints instead. You must let the forearms go down toward the floor or the move becomes too much like the press.

5. THE PULLDOWN

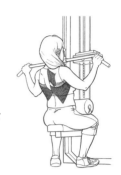

What It's Working

The latissimus dorsi (the muscles along the sides of your back), the upper back, and the rear head of the shoulders.

Do the Move

Sit at a lat pulldown station and grab the bar overhead with an overhand grip, hands slightly wider than shoulder-width apart. Sit down and brace your legs under the kneepads for support. Your arms should naturally be straightened above your head. With your head facing forward and your back straight, slowly pull the bar down to the front of your chest. Slowly let the bar raise your hands back above your head, resisting the pull of the weight as you go, and repeat.

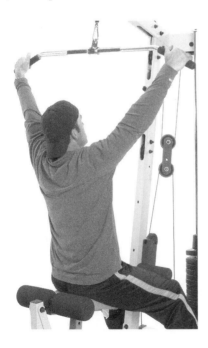

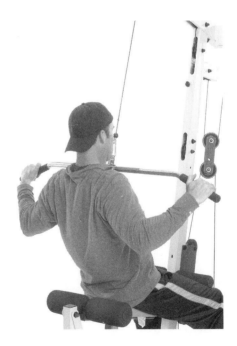

Feel the Move

As you pull the bar down to your chest, roll your shoulders back and gently try to squeeze your shoulder blades together as if someone were taking your coat for you. Your chest should rise slightly as your elbows naturally draw back toward each other behind your back.

The Mistakes Everybody Makes

Don't let the bar yank your arms back overhead. Pulling the bar down to your chest may feel like the only thing that's working your back muscles, but controlling the weight as you bring the bar back overhead works them as well.

Don't pull the bar down past your chest. Pull toward your collarbone (clavicle). Also, it's common to see people pull the bar behind them, but this position rotates your shoulder blades backward and can place unnecessary stress on your tendons.

Finally, don't lean back or arch your spine too much. Arching your back or bending backward too much from your waist brings your smaller lower back muscles into play to help "pull" the bar down.

6. THE ROW

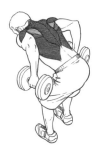

What It's Working

Upper and mid-back muscles, biceps, and the rear head of the shoulders.

Do the Move

Stand straight with a dumbbell in each hand. Bend forward at the waist until your back is almost parallel to the floor, knees bent. Your arms should be hanging down, palms facing each other. Now, keeping your arms close to your torso, pull both dumbbells straight up until they touch the sides of your chest. The motion should resemble rowing. Hold for a second, slowly lower the weights back toward the floor, and repeat.

Feel the Move

Try to forget about everything from the waist down to help you focus on your back muscles. Once you've pulled the weights up as high as you can, imagine that you're trying to bring your elbows close to the center of the body. Concentrating on that posture will align your arms in a way that keeps the back muscles engaged—instead of involving more of your shoulders and biceps—giving your back a more thorough workout. Think about the shoulders rolling toward the rear as if someone were helping you off with your coat—it's the key to keeping the lats engaged.

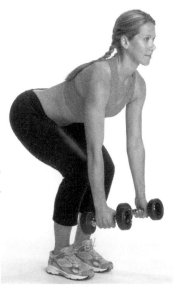
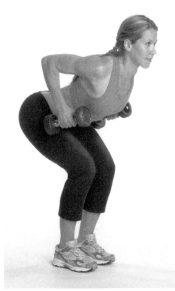

Keep your back as flat as possible. Rounding your spine not only makes it harder to direct the effort of the exercise to the right muscles, but it also makes the exercise more risky.

Don't try using your arms to lift the weight. Trying to pull the weights up with your arms will only exhaust your weaker biceps muscles before your back does its share of the work. Instead, focus on pulling your elbows, not the weights, as high as possible. Think of the arms and hands as hooks attaching the weights to the body. Don't let the energy leak out in an overzealous grip.

7. THE SHOULDER PRESS

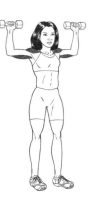

What It's Working

Front and side heads of the shoulders, triceps, and the upper trapezius (the muscles along the neck toward the back).

Do the Move

Stand straight with a dumbbell in each hand. Raise the weights up to the sides of your shoulders, turning your palms so that they face forward. This is the starting position of the move. Slowly press the weights over your head, keeping your back straight as you go. Lower the weights back down to your shoulders and repeat.

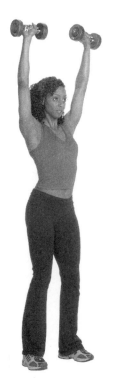
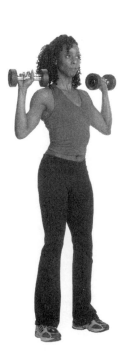

Bend your knees slightly and sink your hips like you're about to absorb a blow. You should feel your shoulders contracting throughout the entire exercise. If you feel less stress on them once your arms are raised, you're probably locking your elbows unintentionally. Relax your grip. Hold the dumbbells only tightly enough to keep control. Anything tighter takes the exercise out of the shoulders and places it in your wrists and hands.

The Mistakes Everybody Makes

Don't pull your arms back behind your body. Some people draw their shoulders back too far. This position actually redirects some of the effort onto the rotator cuff muscles, a series of four tiny stabilizing muscles within the shoulder joint that aid in rotation. Instead, keep your elbows in line with the side of your torso, and don't lower them too far down as that will put excessive strain on the shoulder joint.

Never look up at the weights. Watching the weights rise over your head not only places a strain on your neck, but it can also cause you to lose your balance. Instead, stick with performing the exercise in front of a mirror to check your form.

8. THE RAISE

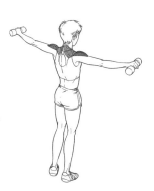

What It's Working

When your torso is vertical, anterior and medial deltoids.
When your torso is horizontal, rear deltoid.

Do the Move

Stand straight with your feet shoulder-width apart holding a light dumbbell in each hand. Your arms should be hanging at your sides, palms facing in toward your thighs. This is the starting position of the move. Slowly raise the weight up with a slight bend in your elbows and out to your sides until your arms are parallel to the floor, palms facing down (You should look like the letter "T".) Hold for a second, slowly lower your arms back down to your sides, and repeat.

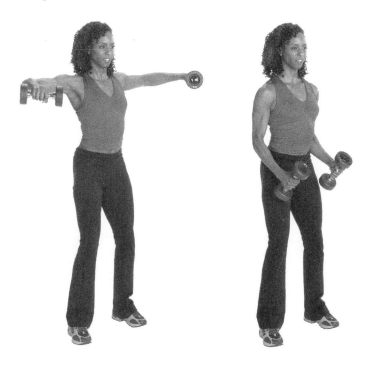

Feel the Move

I tell my clients to imagine themselves as marionettes with strings attached just above their elbows. As you raise the weight, don't think about lifting your hands, but picture having your elbows raised up instead from these strings.

The Mistakes Everybody Makes

Don't let your arms drift forward as you raise the weights. This takes some of the effort off of the sides of your shoulders, dumping all the work on the front of your shoulders.

Try not to bend your elbows more than you have to. You need to keep a slight bend in your arms so that your elbows don't lock, but bending them too much can change how much of your shoulder muscles are engaged throughout the movement.

Once your arms are parallel to the floor (when doing the raise from a vertical position), try rotating your wrists so that the index finger drops slightly below the pinky. Imagine that you're holding two pitchers of water and you're trying to top off someone's glass. This twist stresses the shoulder muscles even further for more results. Lastly, remember that a soft grip is your friend!

9. THE PRESSDOWN

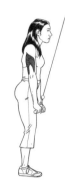

What It's Working

All three heads of the triceps muscles (the muscles along the back of your arms).

Do the Move

Stand facing a high-cable pulley with your back straight and feet shoulder-width apart. Grab the bar with an overhand grip, hands about six to twelve inches apart. Keeping your back straight, tuck your upper arms into your sides and position your forearms so they are parallel to the floor. This is the start of the move. Now, slowly push down the bar until your arms are straight (the bar should be down by and slightly in front of your thighs). Squeeze your triceps for a second, slowly raise the bar back up until your forearms are once again parallel to the floor, and repeat.

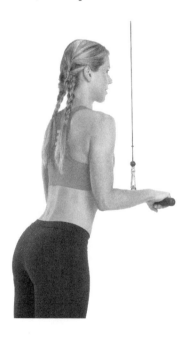
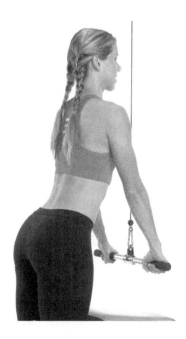

Feel the Move

Don't think about pushing the bar down. Instead, think about pushing it down and "away" so that the bar ends up over your toes. That will keep you from leaning forward onto the bar, which makes it easier to use your shoulders to cheat the weight down. At the bottom of the move (when your arms are straight), tighten your triceps as if someone were about to touch them and you wanted to impress her. (You know you do that!) This helps engage the muscles more fully and also makes sure that you don't release the contraction.

The Mistakes Everybody Makes

Don't let your arms wing out to the sides. This prevents the exercise from working all three heads that make up the triceps muscles, since the angle lets your stronger shoulder muscles help out. Instead, lock your upper arms at your sides. This position keeps all the attention of the exercise focused on the three heads of the triceps while letting you feel your triceps working.

Don't let your elbows lift up. Raising your elbows up means you're lifting your shoulders to push the weight down like you were using a pump to inflate a bike tire. This brings your shoulder and chest muscles and body weight into play to help cheat the weight down.

10. THE EXTENSION

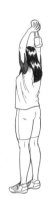

What It's Working

All three heads of the triceps muscles (the muscles along
the back of your arms).

Do the Move

Stand straight with a light dumbbell in your hands and raise it straight above your head.
The dumbbell should hang so that it's vertical, with the top plate resting comfortably on
the palms of your hands, thumbs around the handle. This is the start of the move. Now,
slowly lower the weight behind your head until your forearms are parallel to the floor. Your
elbows should end up pointing toward the ceiling. Slowly raise the weight back over your
head and repeat.

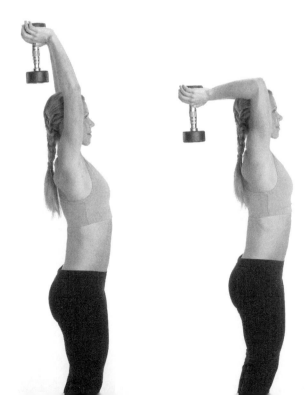

Feel the Move

The move should always feel as if you're pushing the weight "up," never forward. A soft grip, pressing with the heels of your hands, will ensure that the pushing triceps muscles, not the squeezing hand and forearm muscles, are doing the work.

The Mistakes Everybody Makes

Don't grab the weight. Try wrapping the webbing of your hands around the dumbbell so that the bottom of the top part of the dumbbell rests flat on top of your palms. The weight of the dumbbell will hold it in place without wearing out the muscles in your hand. Your elbows should stay pointed toward the ceiling. If they stray forward, the dumbbell will hit you in the back of the head. If you feel that, that's *me* telling *you* that you've let your arms drift too far forward!

11. THE CURL

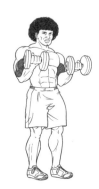

What It's Working

Biceps (the front of your arms) and forearms (the part of your arms below your elbows).

Do the Move

Stand holding a dumbbell in each hand with your arms hanging straight down along your sides or just in front of your quads, palms facing forward. Keeping your elbows tucked into your body, slowly curl the weights up toward your shoulders in a semicircular motion until your forearms touch your biceps. Your palms should end up facing the front of your shoulders. Slowly lower the weights back down until your arms are back down along your sides, palms facing forward, and repeat.

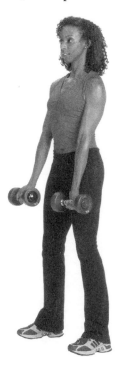
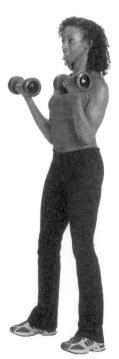

Feel the Move

Throughout the move, your upper arms should stay pinned to your body—as if I've duct-taped you all the way around your body from your elbows to your shoulders. When I'm working with people, I'll hold their upper arms into their sides. I tell them that if they're pushing out against me, they're spending too much energy on that when they should be spending energy curling that weight up.

The Mistakes Everybody Makes

The only things you should ever see moving in the mirror are your lower arms. Most people arch their backs and rock back and forth to help pull the weights up. Instead, pull your upper arms tight into your body and don't move them throughout the entire movement. If they move either forward or backward (instead of being perpendicular to the floor), it means you're most likely cheating the weight up with your lower back.

Don't let your wrists bend backward. Some people let the weight of whatever they're using for resistance pull their wrists downward as they curl. However, bending the wrists backward (or even forward) as you curl shifts some of the stress of the exercise away from the biceps muscles and redistributes it onto your wrist joints—another potential energy leak that you can avoid for better, faster results.

12. THE CRUNCH

What It's Working

The upper portion of your rectus abdominis (the sheet of muscles that make up your abdominals).

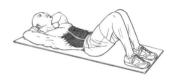

Do the Move

Lie flat on the floor with your knees bent and your feet placed flat on the floor. Place your hands lightly along the sides of your head. This is the starting position. Next, contract your abdominal muscles by pulling them in, then slowly curl your torso forward, raising your head and shoulder blades off the floor. Pause for one second, lower yourself back down to the floor, and repeat.

Feel the Move

Before they start the exercise, I pretend to punch my clients in the stomach to get them to contract, or tense up, in anticipation of the blow. It's that natural reaction of pulling in and contracting your abdominal muscles that should initiate each and every crunch before you even bother to raise yourself off the floor. Also, imagine that you're drawing your ribs up instead of your head and shoulders. The object isn't to "curl" yourself up as much as to "raise" yourself up.

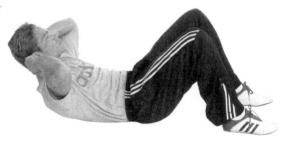

The Mistakes Everybody Makes

Don't raise too high. Your abdominal muscles are involved only within the first forty-five degrees of the movement. Once you raise up past this point, most of the effort of the exercise shifts from your abs to your hip flexors. Instead, try to remember to keep your tailbone on the floor at all times. If you feel your lower back leave the ground, you've raised yourself higher than you need to for the intended abdominal work. There is nothing wrong with going higher from a functional standpoint; it's just not as effective in keeping continuous tension on the abdominals.

Don't lace your hands behind your head. Doing this only makes it easier to pull your head forward and down, placing stress on your neck muscles. Instead, touch your fingers lightly on your head or behind your ears.

You shouldn't ever see your knees. If you're keeping your head in line with your spine, your view will always be looking up and slightly forward. If you can see your kneecaps, you've either raised yourself up too far, tilted your head down too far, or you have really long shins.

Don't let yourself flop back down to the floor. Resisting gravity on the way down will work your abdominal muscles as well, giving you more results from the same exercise. Let yourself drop back to the floor and you'll get less out of it than you could.

13. THE REVERSE CRUNCH

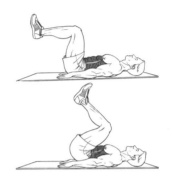

What It's Working

The lower portion of your rectus abdominis.

Do the Move

Lie flat on your back with your arms out to the sides, palms flat to the floor. Keeping your legs together, bend your knees and draw them up until your legs form a ninety-degree angle. Your thighs should be perpendicular to the floor. Next, slowly lift your pelvis off the floor and curl it toward your rib cage. Your knees should automatically curl toward your chest. Pause, then slowly lower your pelvis back down to the floor, keeping your knees up, and repeat.

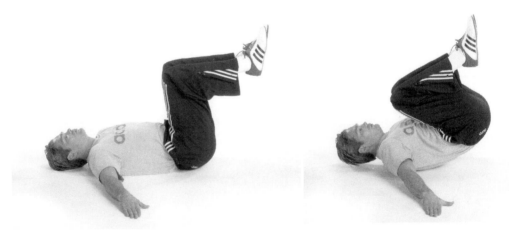

Feel the Move

Don't think about drawing your knees in toward your chest. Instead, imagine you have a glass of water resting just below your belly button. Before you pull your knees in, tilt that glass toward your ribs first. This helps to position your body in a way that teaches you to feel the lower part of your abdominal wall contract. Think about initiating the movement for a backward roll, or even the lower-body portion of a "cannonball" dive into a pool. Relax your ankles! The closer your hands are to your body, the harder it is.

The Mistakes Everybody Makes

Don't move your upper body at all. People see the word *crunch* and their natural inclination is to move their head, shoulders, and torso. Your entire torso from your head to your tailbone should be nailed on the floor as if you were pinned under something heavy.

UNLOCK YOUR FITNESS FREEDOM!

Thirteen exercises. That's it.

You might have expected more from someone who's been a trainer for almost two decades. Well, now that you can do each of the Lucky Thirteen moves with perfect form, I'm going to give you the freedom to work with these classic, performance-proven moves to create fresh, dynamic workouts.

Why would you want to do that? Here comes the good part!

As I mentioned early in this book, your body handles a new exercise plan the same way that you might handle a new job. At first, it's a challenge for you, and you've got to put a lot into getting things done. Eventually, however, you start figuring out how to get your work done faster so you can spend more time surfing the Web, making personal phone calls, and reading the paper. Your work is still getting done, but your progress to that corner office has definitely slowed. Besides being mind-numbingly boring, doing the same fitness routine over and over again has the same effect on your muscles. Your muscles eventually come to know what to expect and learn easier ways to get their jobs done using less effort and burning fewer calories, and, by default, achieving fewer new results.

Some of my clients hate it when they hit a plateau, but I remind them that reaching a plateau in your exercise plan isn't always a bad thing. In fact, hitting that wall can indicate that you're right on track with getting the fitness results you're hoping for. Sticking with a routine long enough to have it slow down on you means you're still sticking to it. Finding the determination to *keep exercising* is the hardest thing for most people, so you've already overcome the biggest obstacle. If you find yourself leveling off, pat yourself on the back. Give yourself some credit for getting there. And don't worry—shaking up your routine will help your body jump back on the road to progress.

Your muscles adapt to stress quickly and learn how to do each exercise with less effort within six to eight workouts. To keep the results coming, you've got to confuse your muscles by changing your routine every three to four weeks, no matter how much you like what you're doing. However, mixing things up doesn't have to mean a complete workout overhaul. Just changing a few variables can be enough to feel different to your muscles. This is one reason many people who train with me never stop improving and one reason why I never stop coming to work.

THE SPIN-OFFS

Figuring out how to create new, challenging exercises isn't as confusing as a lot of trainers try to make it out to be. As I revealed in an earlier chapter, most of the creative exercises you've ever been confused or curious about are merely spin-offs of the Lucky Thirteen. A few subtle tweaks can have a big impact on keeping your body guessing and those fat calories burning.

SPIN-OFF 1: CHANGE YOUR POSTURE

How you position your body during an exercise can significantly change its impact on your muscles. There are a few simple ways you can position your body to affect the angle and get a different effect from an exercise. Here are some of the spin-off postures:

Stand

The perks: I start many of the Lucky Thirteen from this position because it's one of the most practical and functional ways I know to do an exercise. When you need to pull off anything physical during the day, it's often done when you're standing. This position gives you the added benefit of better balance by teaching the rest of your body to work together with the muscles you're actually strengthening during the move.

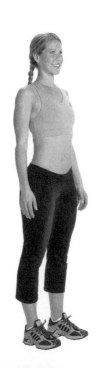

Sit on a Bench (or Chair)

The perks: Sitting down when doing free-weight exercises (like curls or presses) can be a smart way to isolate the muscles you want to work, since it prevents you from using your legs or arching your back to create enough momentum to cheat the weight up. Because it's more difficult to cheat, always pick a weight that's between twenty and twenty-five percent less than what you typically use when doing the exercise from a standing position.

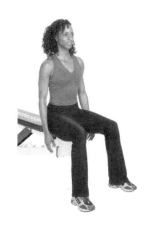

Kneel

The perks: Getting down on your knees can also have the same effect as sitting down, since this posture spin-off makes it harder to cheat with your legs or back.

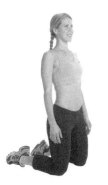

Sit on a Stability Ball

The perks: Using a stability ball is one of the best ways to jump-start your routine. Just positioning yourself on the ball forces all of your muscles (especially the muscles of your core) to naturally contract to stabilize your body in an upright, balanced position before you even start to exercise. This can strengthen your body in a way that's more natural to how your muscles typically work together in real life.

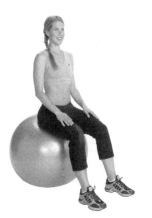

Lie on a Stability Ball

The perks: This spin-off posture offers all the same benefits that sitting on a stability ball does, only it's used more for exercises that typically require you to lie on a mat or bench.

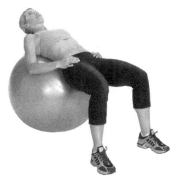

Lie on a Mat

The perks: This posture, used mostly for moves that use your own body weight to work your abdominal muscles, can be done on any mat or even a thick rug.

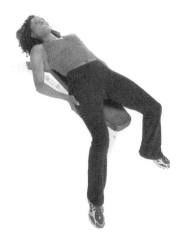

Lie on a Flat Bench

The perks: Used mainly for exercises that require a stable back, this posture also gives you more room so that your elbows can go lower than your body. Try doing the chest press on the floor and you'll feel your elbows touch the ground before you have the chance to lower the weights to the sides of your chest.

Lie on an Incline Bench

The perks: Many benches stay fixed in a flat position, but some allow the backrest to incline. Raising the angle of your torso (from fifteen to forty-five degrees) can change the effect of an exercise, making it focus on different muscle fibers within the same muscles you're trying to develop.

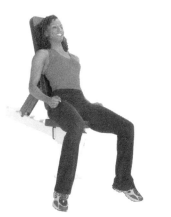

Lie on a Decline Bench

The perks: Some benches also allow the backrest to decline at an angle between thirty and forty-five degrees below parallel. This position offers the same benefits as lying on an incline bench, only inversely.

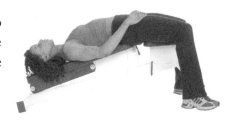

Hang from a Chin-up Bar

The perks: Grabbing a chin-up bar can let you use the weight of your legs and/or upper body as resistance (depending on the exercise).

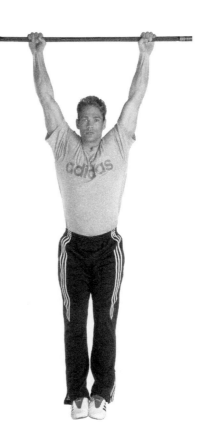

SPIN-OFF 2: CHANGE YOUR TOOLS

When it comes to resistance, your muscles do not judge. All things being equal, they don't know whether it's iron, rubber, cable, or body weight that they're struggling against. All they know is that they're being forced to work harder and become stronger. Still, each tool comes with its own special perks that may be more helpful in certain situations. Here are some of the most common spin-off tools:

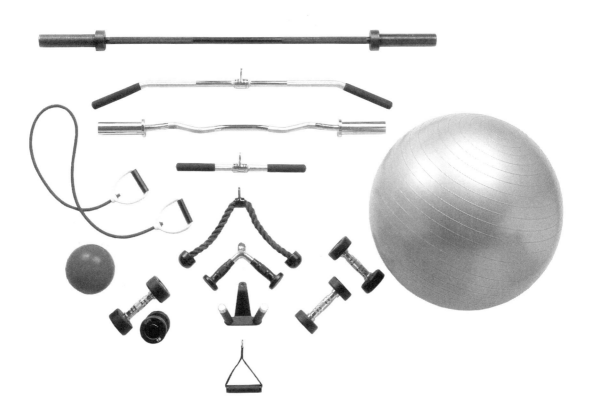

Barbell

The perks: One of the most effective tools for improving muscular strength, a barbell (a long, straight bar that lets you put weight plates on either end or has the plates already attached) allows you to perform hundreds of exercises. You can lift one weight with both hands, which lets you handle heavier loads. This in turn will enable you to get stronger faster than you could by using each hand separately.

E-Z Curl Bar

The perks: With angles at the natural grip placements, this bar angles your wrists as you curl, press (during extensions), or pull (during rows). This tweak can help alleviate excess strain on your wrists, especially when using heavier weights.

Pair of Dumbbells

The perks: Dumbbells (which are actually short versions of barbells, typically ten to fifteen inches in length) offer all the strength-building benefits of a barbell, plus greater versatility in the exercises they can be used for. Lifting two weights with separate hands also prevents your dominant arm from doing more of the work.

Medicine Ball

The perks: These weighted balls come in a variety of weights and sizes, ranging from baseball size to bigger than a basketball. They usually have a softer, textured surface that makes them easy to grip and ideal for pulling off more functional exercises—moves that mimic everyday movements or activities—such as throwing a weight to a partner.

Set of Resistance Bands

The perks: Using resistance bands (or rubber tubing) is like working out with a huge rubber band. Once you secure it to something, you can strengthen your muscles from any angle (using free weights only lets you work your muscles by raising them up and down). You can attach resistance bands anywhere, which lets you pull against them from any and every direction, instead of just fighting against gravity.

This spin-off isn't just ideal for travelers looking to work out on the road. Bands also tend to be easier on your joints than free weights, since the resistance builds gradually as you stretch it. Some brands have handles attached to the ends, and some come with a self-anchoring system that hooks over or onto a door frame so you never have to worry about tying the bands or having anything snap back at you.

High-Cable or Low-Cable Pulley System

The perks: Just like resistance bands, using a pulley system lets you work muscles through a wide variety of angles (instead of just raising a weight straight up and straight down). Plus, you can increase the resistance by adding more weight.

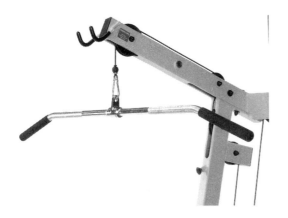 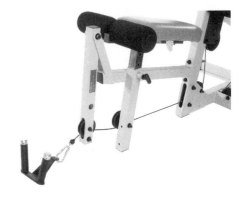

Cable Attachments

The perks: What you attach to a low- or high-cable pulley can change the position of your wrists. The advantage? These new angles will work your muscles in a variety of ways, adding up to a more thorough workout.

Some examples include:

–A lat pulldown bar

–A single-cable handle

–A medium-size straight bar

–An attachable rope, single or double

–A Tri-V bar

–A parallel-grip handle

SPIN-OFF 3: CHANGE YOUR GRIP OR STANCE

Varying the way you hold the bar can shift the stress of an exercise to different sections of the same muscle group, leaving you with a more thoroughly worked muscle that has no choice but to get stronger. To get more results, try out these alternatives.

Wide Grip

As the name implies, you should space your hands a few inches wider than shoulder-width apart.

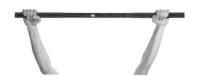

Close Grip

Space your hands about four to twelve inches apart from each other, closer together than you would in normal grip.

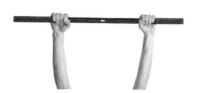

Reverse Grip (Shoulder-Width Apart)

If a Lucky Thirteen exercise normally has you holding the weights with your palms up, then simply turn your wrists inward and flip your hands to grab the weights palms down. If the move has you holding the weights palms down, you'll turn your wrists outward to grab the weight with your palms up. Your hands should still be spaced shoulder-width apart from each other. It's that simple.

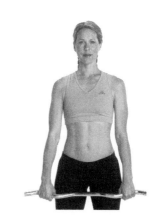

Reverse Wide Grip

For this spin-off, hold the bar in a reverse grip but separate your hands a few inches wider than shoulder-width apart.

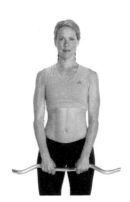

Reverse Close Grip

For this spin-off, hold the bar in reverse grip but keep your hands about four to twelve inches apart from each other.

Palms Facing Toward Each Other

There are a few attachments (such as a parallel-grip handle or a "Double D" handle) that let you do this, but this grip spin-off is typically reserved for when you are holding a set of dumbbells. If the exercise asks for this grip, just keep your hands in the same position as you would while doing the Lucky Thirteen move, but rotate your wrists so they face each other.

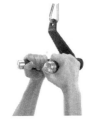

THE NEXT STEP

Now that you understand the Lucky Thirteen and all three spin-off techniques (Posture, Tools, Grip), it's time to show you how to make them all work together.

In this section, I'm going to give you complete freedom. I'm going to show you just *some* of the thousands of possible combinations you can create based on the Lucky Thirteen. I told you that if your muscles aren't constantly challenged, you'll stop seeing results. Well, now you'll have plenty of exercises to choose from—all spun off of the original Lucky Thirteen—when you, or your body, feel it's time for a change (or when someone is using the equipment you need).

Before you get too excited, you have to know something right from the start. You won't be able to change *all* of the Lucky Thirteen exercises using *all* of the different spin-offs. Certain combinations can be more risky, less effective, or simply are impossible to do. Try to do a chest press using dumbbells from a kneeling position and you'll see what I mean. That's called a face plant, and, no, it's not an exercise.

But that's okay. After all, you're about to have nearly a thousand permutations at your disposal.

First, I'll reintroduce you to each of the Lucky Thirteen. Then, I'll show you which posture, tool, and grip spin-offs you can use for each of the thirteen exercises. Finally, instead of having you guess how to combine them all, I've already done some work for you in an easy-to-follow chart.

What you'll see is something that looks like this:

The Lucky Thirteen Move	Posture Spin-Off	Tool Spin-Off	Grip Spin-Off	Here's a Twist	Here's What You've Just Created	Here's What Type of Exercise It Is	Who Should Do It?
Chest press	Lie on a flat bench	Barbell	Normal	N/A	Barbell bench press	Primary or secondary	Level 1–4

Each row starts with the Lucky Thirteen exercise you're looking to change. Keep reading across and you'll see which spin-off postures, tools, and grips you'll need to combine to make a new exercise. After that, you're ready to substitute the new spin-off you've created in place of the original Lucky Thirteen exercise.

The Twist

To give you even more variety, I've added an extra column called "Here's a Twist." Every so often, you'll see that I've tweaked some of the spin-offs. I might ask you to twist the weights as you lift them, twist your body from side to side, or use one leg or one arm at a time. Sometimes, adding these subtle tweaks to an exercise can yield even greater results.

Need a Name for What You're Doing?

To help you keep track of the move I'm referring to, I've given an "official" name to each spin-off we'll create. I use these types of cues with my clients as well.

Who Should Do It?

At the very end of each row, you'll see who can use the spin-off. Most of the moves you're about to create can be used by anyone, regardless of your level of exercise expertise. However, some take a bit more strength, flexibility, or patience than you may have in the early stages of your fitness training. Find where you rank to see which spin-offs you should or shouldn't use before you try any of them as a substitute.

Level 1: Beginning exercisers. If you're new to exercise or have just mastered the Lucky Thirteen, then this means you. Relax. Concentrate on the basics first and you'll be farther down the list in no time.

Level 2: Intermediate exercisers. If you've been doing some form of resistance training consistently for at least two to three months, then you qualify. "Consistently" means you've been weight training at least three days a week for two to three months, not that you joined the gym two to three months ago.

Level 3: Advanced exercisers. You've been dedicated to resistance training for at least one to two years (three to four times a week minimum) before trying a Level 3 spin-off. Remember, just because a spin-off is advanced doesn't mean you'll advance using it if you're not ready.

Level 4: Serious athletes. Some of my most creative, functional moves are best suited for the professional athletes who work with me on a daily basis. There are a few exercises in these charts that can be a huge benefit to the serious exerciser who is active in a sport and has a minimum of two solid years of resistance-training experience. But again, if this isn't you, stick with a lower level. I promise you, the results will never stop coming, and you are much less likely to get injured.

1. SPIN-OFF OF THE SQUAT

Whether you're looking for strong, athletic, full-court-running legs, or the lean, hard legs of A-list actors, these below-the-belt moves will take your legs wherever they need to be.

SPIN-OFF 1: CHANGE YOUR POSTURE

The Lucky Thirteen Posture: Standing

Posture Spin-Off 1: Standing (Against Wall)

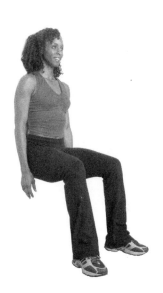

This spin-off makes it easier to keep your balance as you squat by using a sturdy wall to support you. Stand about eighteen inches away from a wall with your back to it. Lean back until your entire back is supported by the wall. Now, slowly lower yourself down, sliding down the wall as you go, until your thighs are parallel to the floor. Push yourself back up the wall. (To help you slide, try placing a towel over your back to start.)

SPIN-OFF 2: CHANGE YOUR TOOLS

The Lucky Thirteen Tool: Barbell

Tool Spin-Off 1: Two Dumbbells

Instead of holding a bar across your shoulders, grab a set of dumbbells. Let your arms hang straight down along your sides with your palms facing in toward your legs. Or just hold the dumbbells at your shoulders.

Tool Spin-Off 2: Medicine Ball

To use this spin-off, hold the medicine ball with both hands in front of your chest.

Since all you're using is your own weight as resistance, just hold your hands at your sides as you squat.

SPIN-OFF 3: CHANGE YOUR GRIP

The Lucky Thirteen Grip: Normal (Hands Shoulder-Width Apart, Pointing Forward)

Grip Spin-Off 1: Palms Facing Each Other

This spin-off comes into play only when you are using dumbbells or holding a medicine ball.

Grip Spin-Off 2: Hold the Weight in Front

Instead of holding the bar across your back, rest the bar across the top of your chest. Cross your arms in front of you and grab the bar with your palms facing in. (This crossed-arm position gives you a more secure grip.) With your back straight, squat down until your thighs are almost parallel to the floor, then stand back up.

When using dumbbells, hold them up by your shoulders as if you were about to do a shoulder press (arms bent, elbows pointing down, and palms facing forward). You can also rest the ends of each dumbbell on the front of your shoulders.

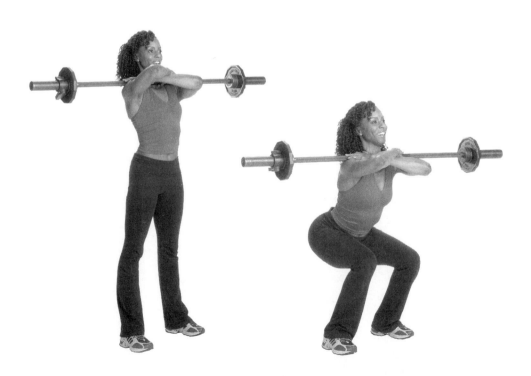

Hold the Ball Overhead

The softness of a medicine ball makes it safer to try this more difficult twist for the squat. Whenever you see it, just extend your arms up over your head so that the ball is directly above you.

Stand on one foot

Some variations that have you leaning against a wall may also suggest standing on one foot. This lets you strengthen your legs separately, in case you have one leg that's stronger than the other and you want to train them individually. To do this, just raise one foot off the floor slightly so that it doesn't help the other leg when you push yourself back up along the wall. This variation can also be done standing without the support of a wall, which involves much more balance.

Rise up! On your toes!

This twist not only helps develop your sense of balance, but also engages your calves (the muscles of the lower leg). Each time you press yourself back into a standing position, rise up a little higher by pushing up on the balls of your feet. This is called a *triple extension* and is an athletic move as it replicates movement in many sports.

READY TO TAKE CHARGE OF YOUR WORKOUTS?

Thought you knew only a handful of exercises to work your legs and calves? Look at what you can do now!

STANDING

The Lucky Thirteen Move	Posture Spin-Off	Tool Spin-Off	Grip Spin-Off	Here's a Twist	Here's What You've Just Created	Here's What Type of Exercise It Is	Who Should Do It?
Squat	Stand	Barbell	Normal	N/A	Barbell squat	Primary or secondary	Level 1–4
Squat	Stand	Barbell	Normal	Rise up on your toes	Barbell squat/ calf raise	Primary or secondary	Level 2–4
Squat	Stand	Barbell	Normal	Hold the weight in front	Front squat	Primary or secondary	Level 2–4
Squat	Stand	Two dumbbells	Palms facing each other	N/A	Dumbbell squat	Primary or secondary	Level 1–4
Squat	Stand	Two dumbbells	Palms facing each other	Rise up on your toes	Dumbbell squat/ calf raise	Primary or secondary	Level 2–4
Squat	Stand	Two dumbbells	Normal	Hold the weight in front	Dumbbell front squat	Primary or secondary	Level 2–4
Squat	Stand	Body weight	N/A	N/A	Body-weight squat	Primary or secondary	Level 1–4
Squat	Stand	Body weight	N/A	Rise up on your toes	Body weight squat/ calf raise	Primary or secondary	Level 2–4
Squat	Stand	Medicine ball	Palms facing each other	N/A	Medicine ball squat	Primary or secondary	Level 1–4
Squat	Stand	Medicine ball	Palms facing each other	Rise up on on your toes	Medicine ball squat/ calf raise	Primary or secondary	Level 2–4
Squat	Stand	Medicine ball	Palms facing each other	Hold the ball overhead	Overhead medicine ball squat	Secondary only	Level 2–4

STANDING AGAINST A WALL

The Lucky Thirteen Move	Posture Spin-Off	Tool Spin-Off	Grip Spin-Off	Here's a Twist	Here's What You've Just Created	Here's What Type of Exercise It Is	Who Should Do It?
Squat	Standing (against wall)	Two dumbbells	Palms facing each other	N/A	Dumbbell wall squat	Primary or secondary	Level 1–4
Squat	Standing (against wall)	Two dumbbells	Palms facing each other	Stand on one foot	One-leg dumbbell wall squat	Primary or secondary	Level 2–4
Squat	Standing (against wall)	Two dumbbells	Rise up on your toes	Palms facing each other	Dumbbell wall squat/ calf raise	Primary or secondary	Level 2–4
Squat	Standing (against wall)	Two dumbbells	Normal	Hold the weight in front	Dumbbell front squat	Primary or secondary	Level 2–4
Squat	Standing (against wall)	Body weight	N/A	N/A	Body-weight wall squat	Primary or secondary	Level 1–4
Squat	Standing (against wall)	Body weight	N/A	Stand on one foot	One-leg body weight wall squat	Primary or secondary	Level 2–4
Squat	Standing (against wall)	Body weight	N/A	Rise up on your toes	Body-weight wall squat/ calf raise	Primary or secondary	Level 2–4
Squat	Standing (against wall)	Medicine ball	Palms facing each other	N/A	Medicine ball wall squat	Primary or secondary	Level 1–4
Squat	Standing (against wall)	Medicine ball	Palms facing each other	Stand on one foot	One-leg medicine ball wall squat	Primary or secondary	Level 2–4
Squat	Standing (against wall)	Medicine ball	Palms facing each other	Rise up on your toes	Medicine ball wall squat/ calf raise	Primary or secondary	Level 2–4
Squat	Standing (against wall)	Medicine ball	Palms facing each other	Hold the ball overhead	Overhead medicine ball wall squat	Secondary only	Level 2–4

2. SPIN-OFF OF THE LUNGE

SPIN-OFF 1: CHANGE YOUR POSTURE

The Lucky Thirteen Posture: Standing (Lunging Backward)

Posture Spin-Off 1: Standing (Lunging Forward)
Instead of stepping backward, you'll be stepping forward. Stand with your back straight and your feet about hip-width apart. Next, step forward as though you were loosely measuring a yard of length with your right leg, bending your right knee so that it stays directly above your ankle and your right thigh is parallel to the floor. Your left heel will naturally lift off the floor as you lunge down. Push yourself back up into a standing position and repeat the move with the left leg.

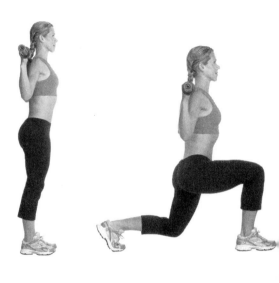

Posture Spin-Off 2: Standing (Lunging to the Side)
Stand straight with your feet together. Take a big step out to the side with your right foot, placing it in line with your left foot. Lean onto your right leg until your thigh is almost parallel to the floor, then push yourself back into a standing position using the right leg. Repeat the move with your left leg.

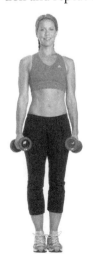

Posture Spin-Off 3: Standing (Lunging Backward and Twisting)

This move is just like the original Lucky Thirteen version of the lunge, only you'll be adding a twist. Stand with your back straight and feet about hip-width apart. This is the start of the move. Take a normal step backward with your right foot, but instead of keeping your right foot facing forward, turn it outward so that it points halfway between out to the side and directly behind you. (If you imagine that your left foot is pointing toward 12 o'clock, your right foot would be pointing toward 4 to 5 o'clock.)

Twist your body to the right as you lunge down with your torso now facing in the same direction as your right knee. Lunge until your right thigh is almost parallel to the floor, then aggressively push yourself back into the starting position, twisting as you go, until you're back in that starting position. Repeat the move, this time stepping back with your left foot.

Posture Spin-Off 4: Standing (Lunging Forward and Reaching)

This move is just like Posture 1, only you'll be reaching down as if you're picking up a small box in front of you. Stand with your back straight and your feet about hip-width apart. Next, take a natural-size step forward with your right leg, slightly bending your right knee so that it's directly above your ankle. Keep the hips high and round the back. This is one of the few times that I will tell you to adopt that rounded back posture. This is a move than we find ourselves doing in real life. If you train for it in the gym, you're less likely to be injured by it in real life. Reach down and extend your hands out toward the floor in front of you as if you were about to pick up a small box. Push yourself back up into a standing position using the right leg and repeat the move with the left leg.

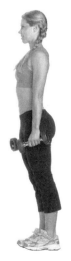
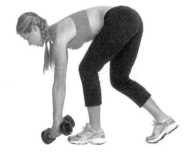

SPIN-OFF 2: CHANGE YOUR TOOLS

The Lucky Thirteen Tool: Barbell

Tool Spin-Off 1: Two Dumbbells

Instead of holding a bar across your shoulders, grab a set of dumbbells. Let your arms hang straight down along your sides with your palms facing in towards your legs.

Tool Spin-Off 2: Medicine Ball

To use this spin-off, hold the medicine ball with both hands in front of your chest (unless I give you a twist).

Tool Spin-Off 3: Your Own Body Weight

Since all you're using is your own weight as resistance, just keep your hands at your sides as you lunge (unless I give you a twist).

Tool Spin-Off 4: One-Hand Low-Cable Pulley

For this spin-off, you'll stand directly in front of a low-cable pulley. Grab the handle with one hand, then step back far enough so that you have room to perform the lunge toward the pulley without letting the weight touch the weightstack. Facing the pulley, perform a lunge toward it until your forward thigh is parallel to the floor (your knee stays over your toes), then push yourself back up into a standing position.

SPIN-OFF 3: CHANGE YOUR GRIP

The Lucky Thirteen Grip: Normal (Hands Shoulder-Width Apart, Pointing Forward)

Grip Spin-Off 1: Palms Facing Each Other

This spin-off comes into play only when using dumbbells or holding a medicine ball.

The Twists to Expect

Place one foot up behind you

This twist challenges your balance while letting you train each leg separately (because most people have one leg that's stronger than the other). Place a sturdy object about two feet high behind you. Extend one leg behind you and rest just the instep of your foot, or your toes, on top of the object (you should now be standing on one leg, with your other leg behind you on the object for balance). Lower your body until your thigh is parallel to the floor, repeat until you finish the desired number of reps, then switch positions to work the opposite leg.

Hold the bar in front of your chest

Instead of holding a barbell behind your neck, you'll hold the barbell in front of you, directly above your chest. When using this twist, remember to reduce the weight you typically use by around twenty-five percent to start.

READY TO TAKE CHARGE OF YOUR WORKOUTS?

Thought you knew only a handful of exercises to work your legs and glutes? Look at what you can do now!

STANDING (LUNGING BACKWARD)

The Lucky Thirteen Move	Posture Spin-Off	Tool Spin-Off	Grip Spin-Off	Here's a Twist	Here's What You've Just Created	Here's What Type of Exercise It Is	Who Should Do It?
Lunge	Stand (lunging backward)	Barbell	Normal	N/A	Reverse barbell lunge	Primary or secondary	Level 1–4
Lunge	Stand (lunging backward)	Two Dumbbells	Palms facing each other	N/A	Reverse dumbbell lunge	Primary or secondary	Level 1–4
Lunge	Stand (lunging backward)	Medicine ball	Palms facing each other	N/A	Reverse medicine ball lunge	Primary or secondary	Level 1–4
Lunge	Stand (lunging backward)	None (body weight)	N/A	N/A	Reverse lunge	Primary or secondary	Level 1–4
Lunge	Stand (lunging backward)	One-hand low-cable pulley	Normal	N/A	Reverse one-arm lunge	Primary or secondary	Level 1–4

STANDING (LUNGING FORWARD)

The Lucky Thirteen Move	Posture Spin-Off	Tool Spin-Off	Grip Spin-Off	Here's a Twist	Here's What You've Just Created	Here's What Type of Exercise It Is	Who Should Do It?
Lunge	Stand (lunging forward)	Barbell	Normal	N/A	Barbell lunge	Primary or secondary	Level 1–4
Lunge	Stand (lunging forward)	Two dumbbells	Palms facing each other	N/A	Dumbbell lunge	Primary or secondary	Level 1–4
Lunge	Stand (lunging forward)	Medicine ball	Palms facing each other	N/A	Medicine ball lunge	Primary or secondary	Level 1–4
Lunge	Stand (lunging forward)	None (body weight)	N/A	N/A	Lunge	Primary or secondary	Level 1–4
Lunge	Stand (lunging forward)	One-hand low-cable pulley	Normal	N/A	One-arm cable Lunge	Primary or secondary	Level 1–4

STANDING (LUNGING TO THE SIDE)

The Lucky Thirteen Move	Posture Spin-Off	Tool Spin-Off	Grip Spin-Off	Here's a Twist	Here's What You've Just Created	Here's What Type of Exercise It Is	Who Should Do It?
Lunge	Stand (lunging to the side)	Barbell	Normal	N/A	Barbell side lunge	Primary or secondary	Level 1–4
Lunge	Stand (lunging to the side)	Two dumbbells	Palms facing each other	N/A	Dumbbell side lunge	Primary or secondary	Level 1–4
Lunge	Stand (lunging to the side)	Medicine ball	Palms facing each other	N/A	Medicine ball side lunge	Primary or secondary	Level 1–4
Lunge	Stand (lunging to the side)	None (body weight)	N/A	N/A	Side lunge	Primary or secondary	Level 1–4
Lunge	Stand (lunging to the side)	One-hand low-cable pulley	Normal	N/A	One-arm side lunge	Primary or secondary	Level 1–4

REACHING LUNGE

The Lucky Thirteen Move	Posture Spin-Off	Tool Spin-Off	Grip Spin-Off	Here's a Twist	Here's What You've Just Created	Here's What Type of Exercise It Is	Who Should Do It?
Lunge	Stand (lunging reaching forward)	Barbell	Normal	Hold the bar in front of your chest	Barbell reaching lunge	Primary or secondary	Level 2–4
Lunge	Stand (lunging reaching forward)	Two dumbbells	Palms facing each other	N/A	Dumbbell reaching lunge	Primary or secondary	Level 2–4
Lunge	Stand (lunging reaching forward)	Medicine ball	Palms facing each other	N/A	Medicine ball reaching lunge	Primary or secondary	Level 2–4
Lunge	Stand (lunging reaching forward)	None (body weight)	N/A	N/A	Reaching lunge	Primary or secondary	Level 2–4
Lunge	Stand (lunging reaching forward)	One-hand low-cable (pulley)	Normal	N/A	One-arm reaching lunge	Primary or secondary	Level 2–4

TWISTING LUNGE

The Lucky Thirteen Move	Posture Spin-Off	Tool Spin-Off	Grip Spin-Off	Here's a Twist	Here's What You've Just Created	Here's What Type of Exercise It Is	Who Should Do It?
Lunge	Stand (lunging turning)	Barbell	Normal	N/A	Barbell twisting lunge	Primary or secondary	Level 2–4
Lunge	Stand (lunging turning)	Two dumbbells	Palms facing each other	N/A	Dumbbell twisting lunge	Primary or secondary	Level 2–4
Lunge	Stand (lunging turning)	Medicine ball	Palms facing each other	N/A	Medicine ball twisting lunge	Primary or secondary	Level 2–4
Lunge	Stand (lunging turning)	None (body weight)	N/A	N/A	Twisting lunge	Primary or secondary	Level 2–4
Lunge	Stand (lunging turning)	One-hand low-cable pulley	Normal	N/A	One-arm twisting lunge	Primary or secondary	Level 2–4

3. SPIN-OFF OF THE CHEST PRESS

SPIN-OFF 1: CHANGE YOUR POSTURE

The Lucky Thirteen Posture: Lie on a Flat Bench

Posture Spin-Off 1: Lie on an Incline Bench

Lie back on an incline bench with a dumbbell in each hand. Raise the weights so they rest along the outside of your chest, palms facing forward. Slowly press the dumbbells straight up above your chest, then lower them back down alongside the sides of your chest.

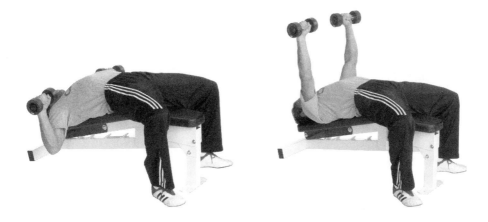

Posture Spin-Off 2: Lie on a Decline Bench

Lie back on a decline bench with a dumbbell in each hand. Raise the weights so they rest along the outside of your chest, palms facing forward. Slowly press the dumbbells straight up above your chest, then lower them back down alongside the sides of your chest.

Posture Spin-Off 3: Lie on a Stability Ball

Sit on a stability ball with your legs bent, feet flat on the floor. Shimmy your feet forward as you slowly roll yourself into a lying position on the ball (just your shoulders and upper back are resting on the ball). With your legs bent at ninety-degree angles for balance (feet flat on the floor), have a partner hand you the weights as you get into position to do the exercise. Press the weight above you, keeping yourself steady on the ball, then lower them back down.

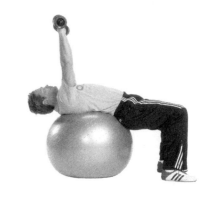

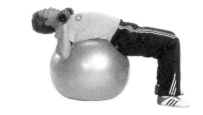

Posture Spin-Off 4: Push-Up Position

Flip yourself over and you can perform the same exercise using your own body weight as resistance. Place your hands flat on the floor (shoulder-width apart) keeping your arms straight, elbows unlocked. Straighten your legs behind you, drawing your feet together. Rise up on your toes. Your body should be one straight line from your heels to your head, your eyes focused straight down at the ground below them. Without moving your head, slowly lower yourself until your upper arms are parallel to the ground, then push yourself back up.

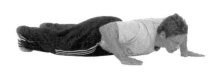

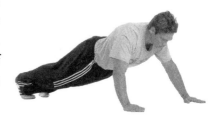

GUNNAR'S TIP

In the charts, you'll see a few variations where you'll be mixing this push-up posture with the tool spin-off of "two dumbbells." All you need to do is place the weights on the floor where you would normally place your hands. Next, grab them as you typically would, then get into a push-up position. Using dumbbells to do push-ups won't add weight to the exercise, but it lets you keep your wrists straight instead of having to bend them. This variation lets you strengthen your forearms while taking some of the wrist stress out of the move.

SPIN-OFF 2: CHANGE YOUR TOOLS

The Lucky Thirteen Tool: Two Dumbbells

Tool Spin-Off 1: Barbell

Tool Spin-Off 2: Resistance Bands

Tool Spin-Off 3: Medicine Ball

You'll be using this tool spin-off only when combined with the push-up posture spin-off. When in a push-up position, you'll place the ball below your chest and place either both hands on the ball or one hand on the ball and one on the floor. Bringing your arms into a narrower position, as you do when using a medicine ball, works more of your inner chest muscles and triceps.

SPIN-OFF 3: CHANGE YOUR GRIP

The Lucky Thirteen Grip: Normal Grip

Grip Spin-Off 1: Wide Grip (Hands Wider Than Shoulder-Width Apart, Overhand Grip, Palms Facing Forward)

Grip Spin-Off 2: Close Grip (Hands Closer Than Shoulder-Width Apart, Overhand Grip, Palms Facing Forward)

Grip Spin-Off 3: Palms Facing Each Other

The Twists to Expect

Twist wrists as you press

If your palms face in toward each other before you start the exercise, you'll twist your wrists inward ninety degrees so they end up facing forward when your arms are overhead. If your palms face forward before you start the exercise, you'll twist your wrists outward ninety degrees so that your palms end up facing each other when your arms are overhead. Either "twist" helps to engage more and different muscle fibers within your chest, not to mention, but I will, that stabilizing the weights while rotating them creates a new challenge for the muscles to adapt to.

Try one arm at a time

Whenever you're asked to do this twist, you'll press one hand up at a time, leaving the other hand down at the side of your chest. This variation isolates each side of your chest by making it harder to use momentum, since you need to go slower just to maintain your balance (plus, the uneven load of one dumbbell requires more core musculature engagement).

Lift up one foot

In *all* of the push-up positions, you can lift one foot just an inch off the floor. This makes it harder to stay balanced as you do the exercise, which forces you to go slower while displacing more of the weight onto your arms for more of a workout. And again, you'll get more of a core workout this way.

Put your feet up

In *all* of the push-up positions, you can place your feet up on a sturdy surface that's between six and twenty-four inches high, or higher (like a step or a small box). This makes the exercise more challenging by shifting more of your body weight forward onto your arms.

READY TO TAKE CHARGE OF YOUR WORKOUTS?

Thought you knew only a handful of exercises to work your chest? Look at what you can do now!

The Lucky Thirteen Move	Posture Spin-Off	Tool Spin-Off	Grip Spin-Off	Here's a Twist	Here's What You've Just Created	Here's What Type of Exercise It Is	Who Should Do It?
Chest press	Lie on a flat bench	Barbell	Normal	N/A	Barbell bench press	Primary or secondary	Level 1–4
Chest press	Lie on a flat bench	Barbell	Wide	N/A	Wide-grip barbell bench press	Primary or secondary	Level 3–4
Chest press	Lie on a flat bench	Barbell	Close	N/A	Close-grip barbell bench press	Secondary only	Level 3–4
Chest press	Lie on a flat bench	Two dumbbells	Normal	N/A	Dumbbell bench press	Primary or secondary	Level 1–4
Chest press	Lie on a flat bench	Two dumbbells	Normal	Twist wrists as you press	Twisting dumbbell bench press	Primary or secondary	Level 1–4
Chest press	Lie on a flat bench	Two dumbbells	Normal	Try one arm at a time	One-arm dumbbell bench press	Primary or secondary	Level 2–4
Chest press	Lie on a flat bench	Two dumbbells	Palms facing each other	N/A	Parallel-grip dumbbell bench press	Primary or secondary	Level 1–4
Chest press	Lie on a flat bench	Two dumbbells	Palms facing each other	Twist wrists as you press	Parallel-grip twisting dumbbell bench press	Primary or secondary	Level 1–4
Chest press	Lie on a flat bench	Two dumbbells	Palms facing each other	Try one arm at a time	One-arm parallel-grip dumbbell bench press	Primary or secondary	Level 2–4
Chest press	Lie on a flat bench	Resistance bands	Normal	N/A	Stretch cord bench press	Primary or secondary	Level 1–4
Chest press	Lie on a flat bench	Resistance bands	Normal	Try one arm at a time	One-arm stretch cord bench press	Primary or secondary	Level 2–4
Chest press	Lie on a flat bench	Resistance bands	Palms facing each other	N/A	Parallel-grip stretch cord bench press	Primary or secondary	Level 1–4

LYING ON AN INCLINE BENCH

The Lucky Thirteen Move	Posture Spin-Off	Tool Spin-Off	Grip Spin-Off	Here's a Twist	Here's What You've Just Created	Here's What Type of Exercise It Is	Who Should Do It?
Chest press	Lie on an incline bench	Barbell	Normal	N/A	Barbell incline bench press	Primary or secondary	Level 1–4
Chest press	Lie on an incline bench	Barbell	Wide	N/A	Wide-grip barbell incline bench press	Primary or secondary	Level 3–4
Chest press	Lie on an incline bench	Barbell	Close	N/A	Close-grip barbell incline bench press	Secondary only	Level 3–4
Chest press	Lie on an incline bench	Two dumbbells	Normal	N/A	Dumbbell incline bench press	Primary or secondary	Level 1–4
Chest press	Lie on an incline bench	Two dumbbells	Normal	Twist wrists as you press	Twisting dumbbell incline bench press	Primary or secondary	Level 1–4
Chest press	Lie on an incline bench	Two dumbbells	Normal	Try one arm at a time	One-arm dumbbell incline bench press	Primary or secondary	Level 2–4
Chest press	Lie on an incline bench	Two dumbbells	Palms facing each other	N/A	Parallel-grip dumbbell incline bench press	Primary or secondary	Level 1–4
Chest press	Lie on an incline bench	Two dumbbells	Palms facing each other	Twist wrists as you press	Parallel-grip twisting dumbbell incline bench press	Primary or secondary	Level 1–4
Chest press	Lie on an incline bench	Two dumbbells	Palms facing each other	Try one arm at a time	One-arm parallel-grip dumbbell incline bench press	Primary or secondary	Level 2–4
Chest press	Lie on an incline bench	Resistance bands	Normal	N/A	Stretch cord incline bench press	Primary or secondary	Level 1–4
Chest press	Lie on an incline bench	Resistance bands	Normal	Try one arm at a time	One-arm stretch cord incline bench press	Primary or secondary	Level 2–4
Chest press	Lie on an incline bench	Resistance bands	Palms facing each other	N/A	Parallel-grip stretch cord incline bench press	Primary or secondary	Level 1–4

The Lucky Thirteen Move	Posture Spin-Off	Tool Spin-Off	Grip Spin-Off	Here's a Twist	Here's What You've Just Created	Here's What Type of Exercise It Is	Who Should Do It?
Chest press	Lie on a decline bench	Barbell	Normal	N/A	Barbell decline bench press	Primary or secondary	Level 1–4
Chest press	Lie on a decline bench	Barbell	Wide	N/A	Wide-grip barbell decline bench press	Primary or secondary	Level 3–4
Chest press	Lie on a decline bench	Barbell	Close	N/A	Close-grip barbell decline bench press	Secondary only	Level 3–4
Chest press	Lie on a decline bench	Two dumbbells	Normal	N/A	Dumbbell decline bench press	Primary or secondary	Level 1–4
Chest press	Lie on a decline bench	Two dumbbells	Normal	Twist wrists as you press	Twisting dumbbell decline bench press	Primary or secondary	Level 1–4
Chest press	Lie on a decline bench	Two dumbbells	Normal	Try one arm at a time	One-arm dumbbell decline bench press	Primary or secondary	Level 2–4
Chest press	Lie on a decline bench	Two dumbbells	Palms facing each other	N/A	Parallel-grip dumbbell decline bench press	Primary or secondary	Level 1–4
Chest press	Lie on a decline bench	Two dumbbells	Palms facing each other	Twist wrists as you press	Parallel-grip twisting dumbbell decline bench press	Primary or secondary	Level 1–4
Chest press	Lie on a decline bench	Two dumbbells	Palms facing each other	Try one arm at a time	One-arm parallel-grip dumbbell decline bench press	Primary or secondary	Level 2–4
Chest press	Lie on a decline bench	Resistance bands	Normal	N/A	Stretch cord decline bench press	Primary or secondary	Level 1–4
Chest press	Lie on a decline bench	Resistance bands	Normal	Try one arm at a time	One-arm stretch cord decline bench press	Primary or secondary	Level 2–4
Chest press	Lie on a decline bench	Resistance bands	Palms facing each other	N/A	Parallel-grip stretch cord decline bench press	Primary or secondary	Level 1–4

LYING ON A STABILITY BALL

The Lucky Thirteen Move	Posture Spin-Off	Tool Spin-Off	Grip Spin-Off	Here's a Twist	Here's What You've Just Created	Here's What Type of Exercise It Is	Who Should Do It?
Chest press	Lie on a ball	Barbell	Normal	N/A	Barbell stability ball bench chest press	Primary or secondary	Level 1–4
Chest press	Lie on a ball	Barbell	Wide	N/A	Wide-grip barbell stability ball chest press	Primary or secondary	Level 3–4
Chest press	Lie on a ball	Barbell	Close	N/A	Close-grip barbell stability ball chest press	Secondary only	Level 3–4
Chest press	Lie on a ball	Two dumbbells	Normal	N/A	Dumbbell stability ball chest press	Primary or secondary	Level 1–4
Chest press	Lie on a ball	Two dumbbells	Normal	Twist wrists as you press	Twisting dumbbell stability ball chest press	Primary or secondary	Level 1–4
Chest press	Lie on a ball	Two dumbbells	Normal	Try one arm at a time	One-arm dumbbell stability ball chest press	Primary or secondary	Level 2–4
Chest press	Lie on a ball	Two dumbbells	Palms facing each other	N/A	Parallel-grip dumbbell stability ball chest press	Primary or secondary	Level 1–4
Chest press	Lie on a ball	Two dumbbells	Palms facing each other	Twist wrists as you press	Parallel-grip twisting dumbbell stability ball chest press	Primary or secondary	Level 1–4
Chest press	Lie on a ball	Two dumbbells	Palms facing each other	Try one arm at a time	One-arm parallel-grip dumbbell stability ball chest press	Primary or secondary	Level 2–4
Chest press	Lie on a ball	Resistance bands	Normal	N/A	Stretch cord stability ball chest press	Primary or secondary	Level 1–4
Chest press	Lie on a ball	Resistance bands	Normal	Try one arm at a time	One-arm stretch cord stability ball chest press	Primary or secondary	Level 2–4
Chest press	Lie on a ball	Resistance bands	Palms facing each other	N/A	Parallel-grip stretch cord stability ball chest press	Primary or secondary	Level 1–4

The Lucky Thirteen Move	Posture Spin-Off	Tool Spin-Off	Grip Spin-Off	Here's a Twist	Here's What You've Just Created	Here's What Type of Exercise It Is	Who Should Do It?
Chest press	Push-up position	N/A	Normal	N/A	Push-up	Primary or secondary	Level 1–4
Chest press	Push-up position	N/A	Wide	N/A	Wide-grip push-up	Primary or secondary	Level 2–4
Chest press	Push-up position	N/A	Close	N/A	Close-grip push-up	Primary or secondary	Level 2–4
Chest press	Push-up position	Two dumbbells	Normal	N/A	Dumbbell push-up	Primary or secondary	Level 1–4
Chest press	Push-up position	Two dumbbells	Wide	N/A	Wide-grip dumbbell push-up	Primary or secondary	Level 3–4
Chest press	Push-up position	Two dumbbells	Close	N/A	Close-grip dumbbell push-up	Primary or secondary	Level 3–4
Chest press	Push-up position	Two dumbbells	Palms facing each other	N/A	Parallel-grip dumbbell push-up	Primary or secondary	Level 2–4
Chest press	Push-up position	Medicine ball	Close	N/A	Medicine ball push-up	Primary or secondary	Level 3–4
Chest press	Push-up position	Medicine ball	Palms facing each other	N/A	Parallel-grip medicine ball push-up	Primary or secondary	Level 3–4
Chest press	Push-up position	Stability ball	Close	N/A	Stability ball push-up	Primary or secondary	Level 3–4
Chest press	Push-up position	Any of the above variations	Any of the above variations	Place your feet up	Elevated push-up	Primary or secondary	Level 2–4
Chest press	Push-up position	Any of the above variations	Any of the above variations	Go on one foot	Unilateral push-up	Primary or secondary	Level 2–4

4. SPIN-OFF OF THE CHEST FLY

SPIN-OFF 1: CHANGE YOUR POSTURE

The Lucky Thirteen Posture: Lie on a Flat Bench

Posture Spin-Off 1: Lie on an Incline Bench

Lie back on an incline bench with a dumbbell in each hand. Extend your arms straight up above your chest, palms facing each other. Bend your elbows slightly, then slowly lower the dumbbells out to your sides in a semicircular arc until they're as low as comfortably possible. Now slowly bring them back together above your chest, using the same semicircular arc.

Posture Spin-Off 2: Lie on a Decline Bench

Lie back on a decline bench with a dumbbell in each hand. Perform the exercise in the same way as you would for the incline bench.

Posture Spin-Off 3: Lie on a Stability Ball

Lie back on a stability ball so that your upper back and shoulder blades rest on top. Your legs should be bent, with your feet flat on the floor to keep yourself stable. Have a partner hand you your weights (or whichever tool you're using with the move), find your balance on the ball, and perform the exercise.

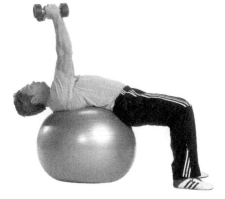
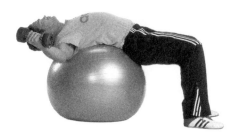

For this posture spin-off, you'll need a cable crossover machine with two pulley stations. Stand between the two cable pulley towers with your feet about shoulder-width apart. Reach and grab one pulley handle from each side in each hand. Now, keeping elbows slightly bent, slowly pull both handles across your body as if you were giving someone a bear hug. Finish the move with your hands outstretched in front of you, knuckles touching. Slowly bring your arms back out to your sides and repeat. Varying the height at which you set the cables can give you even more variations from this spin-off.

SPIN-OFF 2: CHANGE YOUR TOOLS

The Lucky Thirteen Tool: Two Dumbbells

Tool Spin-Off 1: One-Hand Low-Cable Pulley

For any exercise that asks you to use a one-hand low-cable pulley, you'll be placing either a bench, ball, or just yourself between two low-cable pulleys. (In a gym, they call this machine a cable crossover station.) Grab a handle in each hand so that your arms extend out from your sides. As you do the fly, pull your arms up and forward until they're straight in front of your chest (unless you are doing a twist).

Tool Spin-Off 2: One-Hand High-Cable Pulley

Using a set of high-cable pulleys works the same mechanically as the low-cable pulley, only instead of just having your arms extend out from your sides, you'll notice they are raised higher than your shoulders because of the pulley system. That's okay. As you do the fly, pull your arms down and forward until they're straight in front of your chest (unless you are doing a twist). The difference is that the angle in which the muscle is stressed recruits different fibers.

Tool Spin-Off 3: Resistance Bands

For any lying exercises, you'll need to attach the bands about two feet to either side of the bench (ball, etc.) so that you can have resistance coming from the left and right side of you as you perform the fly. For the standing exercises that use resistance bands, stand with both feet on top of the piece of tubing, with your back straight and your feet slightly wider than shoulder-width apart. Grasp the ends of the tubing in both hands and extend both arms out to your sides so that you feel the tension in the tubing. Next, draw your arms together in front of your chest, then slowly return to the starting position.

SPIN-OFF 3: CHANGE YOUR GRIP

The Lucky Thirteen Grip: Palms Facing Each Other

Grip Spin-Off 1: Normal Grip (Overhand Grip, Palms Facing Forward in Front of You)

The Twists to Expect

Twist wrists as you fly

If your palms face in toward each other before you start the exercise, you'll twist your wrists inward ninety degrees so they end up facing forward when your arms are overhead. If your palms face forward before you start the exercise, you'll twist your wrists outward ninety degrees so that your palms end up facing each other when your arms are overhead. Either "twist" helps to engage more of the muscle fibers within your chest.

Try one arm at a time

Whenever you're asked to do this twist, you'll perform the exercise using only one arm. You can place your other hand on your leg or grab the edge of a bench for stability. This variation isolates each side of your chest by making it harder to use momentum, since you need to go slower just to maintain your balance. It also forces your core to work harder to stabilize your body.

Draw your hands below your belt

Some of the standing variations will have you sweep your arms down so that your hands end up below your belt instead of in front of your chest. This works more of the lower portion of your chest muscles.

READY TO TAKE CHARGE OF YOUR WORKOUTS?

Thought you knew only a handful of exercises to work your chest? Look at what you can do now!

The Lucky Thirteen Move	Posture Spin-Off	Tool Spin-Off	Grip Spin-Off	Here's a Twist	Here's What You've Just Created	Here's What Type of Exercise It Is	Who Should Do It?
Chest fly	Lie on a flat bench	Two dumbbells	Palms facing each other	N/A	Chest fly	Primary or secondary	Level 1–4
Chest fly	Lie on a flat bench	Two dumbbells	Palms facing each other	Twist wrists as you fly	Twisting fly	Primary or secondary	Level 1–4
Chest fly	Lie on a flat bench	Two dumbbells	Normal	N/A	Dumbbell chest fly	Primary or secondary	Level 2–4
Chest fly	Lie on a flat bench	Two dumbbells	Normal	Twist wrists as you fly	Dumbbell twisting fly	Primary or secondary	Level 2–4
Chest fly	Lie on a flat bench	One-hand low-cable pulley	Palms facing each other	N/A	Cable fly	Primary or secondary	Level 1–4
Chest fly	Lie on a flat bench	One-hand low-cable pulley	Palm facing in	Try one arm at a time	Unilateral cable fly	Primary or secondary	Level 2–4
Chest fly	Lie on a flat bench	Resistance bands	Palms facing each other	N/A	Stretch cord fly	Primary or secondary	Level 1–4
Chest fly	Lie on a flat bench	Resistance bands	Palm facing in	Try one arm at a time	Unilateral stretch cord fly	Primary or secondary	Level 2–4

LYING ON AN INCLINE BENCH

The Lucky Thirteen Move	Posture Spin-Off	Tool Spin-Off	Grip Spin-Off	Here's a Twist	Here's What You've Just Created	Here's What Type of Exercise It Is	Who Should Do It?
Chest fly	Lie on an incline bench	Two dumbbells	Palms facing each other	N/A	Incline fly	Primary or secondary	Level 1–4
Chest fly	Lie on an incline bench	Two dumbbells	Palms facing each other	Twist wrists as you fly	Incline twisting fly	Primary or secondary	Level 1–4
Chest fly	Lie on an incline bench	Two dumbbells	Normal	N/A	Dumbbell incline fly	Primary or secondary	Level 2–4
Chest fly	Lie on an incline bench	Two dumbbells	Normal	Twist wrists as you fly	Dumbbell twisting incline fly	Primary or secondary	Level 2–4
Chest fly	Lie on an incline bench	One-hand low-cable pulley	Palms facing each other	N/A	Incline cable fly	Primary or secondary	Level 1–4
Chest fly	Lie on an incline bench	One-hand low-cable pulley	Palm facing in	Try one arm at a time	Unilateral incline cable fly	Primary or secondary	Level 2–4
Chest fly	Lie on an incline bench	Resistance bands	Palms facing each other	N/A	Incline stretch cord fly	Primary or secondary	Level 1–4
Chest fly	Lie on an incline bench	Resistance bands	Palm facing in	Try one arm at a time	Unilateral incline stretch cord fly	Primary or secondary	Level 2–4

LYING ON A DECLINE BENCH

The Lucky Thirteen Move	Posture Spin-Off	Tool Spin-Off	Grip Spin-Off	Here's a Twist	Here's What You've Just Created	Here's What Type of Exercise It Is	Who Should Do It?
Chest fly	Lie on a decline bench	Two dumbbells	Palms facing each other	N/A	Decline fly	Primary or secondary	Level 1–4
Chest fly	Lie on a decline bench	Two dumbbells	Palms facing each other	Twist wrists as you fly	Decline twisting fly	Primary or secondary	Level 1–4
Chest fly	Lie on a decline bench	Two dumbbells	Normal	N/A	Dumbbell decline fly	Primary or secondary	Level 2–4
Chest fly	Lie on a decline bench	Two dumbbells	Normal	Twist wrists as you fly	Dumbbell twisting decline fly	Primary or secondary	Level 2–4
Chest fly	Lie on a decline bench	One-hand low-cable pulley	Palms facing each other	N/A	Decline cable fly	Primary or secondary	Level 1–4
Chest fly	Lie on a decline bench	One-hand low-cable pulley	Palm facing in	Try one arm at a time	Unilateral decline cable fly	Primary or secondary	Level 2–4
Chest fly	Lie on a decline bench	Resistance bands	Palms facing each other	N/A	Decline stretch cord fly	Primary or secondary	Level 1–4
Chest fly	Lie on a decline bench	Resistance bands	Palm facing in	Try one arm at a time	Unilateral decline stretch cord fly	Primary or secondary	Level 2–4

LYING ON A STABILITY BALL

The Lucky Thirteen Move	Posture Spin-Off	Tool Spin-Off	Grip Spin-Off	Here's a Twist	Here's What You've Just Created	Here's What Type of Exercise It Is	Who Should Do It?
Chest fly	Lie on a ball	Two dumbbells	Palms facing each other	N/A	Stability ball fly	Primary or secondary	Level 2–4
Chest fly	Lie on a ball	Two dumbbells	Palms facing each other	Twist wrists as you fly	Stability ball twisting fly	Primary or secondary	Level 2–4
Chest fly	Lie on a ball	Two dumbbells	Normal	N/A	Dumbbell stability ball fly	Primary or secondary	Level 2–4
Chest fly	Lie on a ball	Two dumbbells	Normal	Twist wrists as you fly	Dumbbell twisting stability ball fly	Primary or secondary	Level 2–4
Chest fly	Lie on a ball	One-hand low-cable pulley	Palms facing each other	N/A	Stability ball cable fly	Primary or secondary	Level 2–4
Chest fly	Lie on a ball	One-hand low-cable pulley	Palm facing in	Try one arm at a time	Unilateral stability ball cable fly	Primary or secondary	Level 2–4
Chest fly	Lie on a ball	Resistance bands	Palms facing each other	N/A	Stability ball stretch cord fly	Primary or secondary	Level 2–4
Chest fly	Lie on a ball	Resistance bands	Palm facing in	Try one arm at a time	Unilateral stability ball stretch cord fly	Primary or secondary	Level 2–4

STANDING

The Lucky Thirteen Move	Posture Spin-Off	Tool Spin-Off	Grip Spin-Off	Here's a Twist	Here's What You've Just Created	Here's What Type of Exercise It Is	Who Should Do It?
Chest fly	Stand	One-hand high-cable pulley	Normal	N/A	Unilateral chest-level standing high-cable fly	Primary or secondary	Level 1–4
Chest fly	Stand	One-hand high-cable pulley	Palms facing in (face down)	Draw your hands below your belt	Unilateral standing high-cable pullover	Primary or secondary	Level 1–4
Chest fly	Stand	One-hand high-cable pulley	Palms facing in (face down)	Draw one arm down below your belt	Unilateral standing high-cable pullover	Primary or secondary	Level 2–4
Chest fly	Stand	One-hand low-cable pulley	Normal	N/A	Unilateral standing low-cable fly	Primary or secondary	Level 1–4
Chest fly	Stand	One-hand low-cable pulley	Normal	Draw your hands below your belt	Unilateral standing low-cable pullover	Primary or secondary	Level 1–4
Chest fly	Stand	One-hand low-cable pulley	Palm facing in	Try one arm at a time	Standing unilateral low-cable fly	Primary or secondary	Level 2–4
Chest fly	Stand	Resistance bands	Normal	N/A	Standing stretch cord fly	Primary or secondary	Level 1–4
Chest fly	Stand	Resistance bands	Normal	Try one arm at a time	Standing unilateral stretch cord fly	Primary or secondary	Level 1–4

5. SPIN-OFF OF THE PULLDOWN

SPIN-OFF 1: CHANGE YOUR POSTURE

The Lucky Thirteen Posture: Sitting on a Bench

Posture Spin-Off 1: Seated on a Stability Ball

Place a stability ball in front of a high-cable pulley and sit down on the ball facing the cable station. Reach up and grab the bar so that your arms extend over your head. Maintain your balance on the ball, then slowly pull the bar down to the top of your chest.

Posture Spin-Off 2: Standing

This stance spin-off isn't for everyone, especially if you're too tall. But standing can keep your back muscles contracting by limiting the range of motion of the exercise. To do it, stand facing the high pulley and grab the bar with your hands wider than shoulder-width. Your arms won't completely extend over your head; just bend them like you would as if you were pulling the weight. Pull the bar down to your chest, then raise it back up until you can't go any farther.

Posture Spin-Off 3: Kneeling

Stand facing a high-cable pulley and kneel down in front of it. Reach up and grab the bar so that your arms extend over your head. Keeping your head and back straight, slowly pull the bar down to the top of your chest. You will notice a lot of core work with this posture.

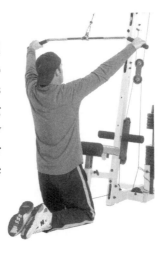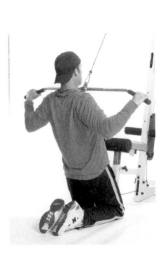

Posture Spin-Off 4: Hanging from a Pull-Up Bar

For this stance spin-off, you won't be using anything but your own body weight as resistance. Doing a "pull-up" works your back muscles in the same exact way that a "pull-down" does. Hang from the bar with your hands shoulder-width apart, legs straight. Slowly, but with conviction, pull yourself up until the bar is under your chin, lower yourself back down and repeat. If you can't even do one at first, work on it and stick with the other exercises. When you finally do one, you will be exhilarated!

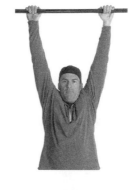

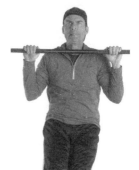

SPIN-OFF 2: CHANGE YOUR TOOLS

**The Lucky Thirteen Tool:
Two-Hand High-Cable Pulley**

Tool Spin-Off 1: One-Hand High-Cable Pulley

For this spin-off, you'll be using a single-cable handle, unless I give you a twist. As you do the exercise, pull your hand down to the side of your chest.

Tool Spin-Off 2. Resistance Bands

For this spin-off, you can loop the middle of the stretch cord over a chin-up bar, the edge of a door, or anything high enough to let you grab both ends and pull them down with resistance.

SPIN-OFF 3: CHANGE YOUR GRIP

The Lucky Thirteen Grip: Wide Grip (Hands Wider Than Shoulder-Width Apart, Overhand Grip, Palms Facing Forward)

Grip Spin-Off 1: Normal Grip (Hands Shoulder-Width Apart, Overhand Grip)

Grip Spin-Off 2: Reverse Grip (Hands Shoulder-Width Apart, Underhand Grip, Palms Facing Backward)

Grip Spin-Off 3: Reverse Close Grip (Hands Closer Than Shoulder-Width Apart, Underhand Grip)

Grip Spin-Off 4: Palms Facing Each Other

To do this spin-off, you'll need a parallel-grip handle or a "Double D" handle attachment.

The Twists to Expect

Attach a rope to the pulley

Hooking a rope (or threading a towel through the pulley clip and grabbing both ends) will let you do the exercise with your palms facing each other. As you pull, try to bring your hands down to the sides of your chest.

READY TO TAKE CHARGE OF YOUR WORKOUTS?

Thought you knew only a handful of exercises to work your back? Look at what you can do now!

The Lucky Thirteen Move	Posture Spin-Off	Tool Spin-Off	Grip Spin-Off	Here's a Twist	Here's What You've Just Created	Here's What Type of Exercise It Is	Who Should Do It?
Pulldown	Sit on a bench	Two-hand high-cable pulley	Normal	N/A	Lat pulldown	Primary or secondary	Level 1–4
Pulldown	Sit on a bench	Two-hand high-cable pulley	Wide	N/A	Wide-grip pulldown	Primary or secondary	Level 1–4
Pulldown	Sit on a bench	Two-hand high-cable pulley	Reverse	N/A	Reverse-grip pulldown	Secondary only	Level 1–4
Pulldown	Sit on a bench	Two-hand high-cable pulley	Reverse close grip	N/A	Reverse close-grip pulldown	Primary or secondary	Level 1–4
Pulldown	Sit on a bench	Two-hand high-cable pulley	Palms facing each other	N/A	Neutral-grip pulldown	Primary or secondary	Level 1–4
Pulldown	Sit on a bench	Two-hand high-cable pulley	Palms facing each other	Attach a rope to the pulley	Rope pulldown	Primary or secondary	Level 2–4
Pulldown	Sit on a bench	One-hand high-cable pulley	Normal	N/A	One-arm pulldown	Primary or secondary	Level 1–4
Pulldown	Sit on a bench	One-hand high-cable pulley	Reverse	N/A	One-arm reverse-grip pulldown	Secondary only	Level 1–4
Pulldown	Sit on a bench	One-hand high-cable pulley	Palm facing in	N/A	One-arm neutral-grip pulldown	Primary or secondary	Level 1–4
Pulldown	Sit on a bench	One-hand high-cable pulley	Palm facing in	Attach a rope to the pulley	One-arm rope pulldown	Primary or secondary	Level 1–4
Pulldown	Sit on a bench	Resistance bands	Normal	N/A	Stretch cord pulldown	Primary or secondary	Level 1–4
Pulldown	Sit on a bench	Resistance bands	Reverse	N/A	Reverse-grip stretch cord pulldown	Secondary only	Level 1–4
Pulldown	Sit on a bench	Resistance bands	Reverse close grip	N/A	Close-grip stretch cord pulldown	Primary or secondary	Level 1–4
Pulldown	Sit on a bench	Resistance bands	Palms facing each other	N/A	Neutral-grip stretch cord pulldown	Primary or secondary	Level 1–4

SITTING ON A STABILITY BALL

The Lucky Thirteen Move	Posture Spin-Off	Tool Spin-Off	Grip Spin-Off	Here's a Twist	Here's What You've Just Created	Here's What Type of Exercise It Is	Who Should Do It?
Pulldown	Sit on a ball	Two-hand high-cable pulley	Normal	N/A	Stability ball pulldown	Primary or secondary	Level 1–4
Pulldown	Sit on a ball	Two-hand high-cable pulley	Wide	N/A	Wide-grip stability ball pulldown	Primary or secondary	Level 1–4
Pulldown	Sit on a ball	Two-hand high-cable pulley	Reverse	N/A	Reverse-grip stability ball pulldown	Secondary only	Level 1–4
Pulldown	Sit on a ball	Two-hand high-cable pulley	Reverse close grip	N/A	Close-grip stability ball pulldown	Primary or secondary	Level 1–4
Pulldown	Sit on a ball	Two-hand high-cable pulley	Palms facing each other	N/A	Neutral-grip stability ball pulldown	Primary or secondary	Level 1–4
Pulldown	Sit on a ball	Two-hand high-cable pulley	Palms facing each other	Attach a rope to the pulley	Rope stability ball pulldown	Primary or secondary	Level 1–4
Pulldown	Sit on a ball	One-hand high-cable pulley	Normal	N/A	One-arm stability ball pulldown	Primary or secondary	Level 1–4
Pulldown	Sit on a ball	One-hand high-cable pulley	Reverse	N/A	One-arm reverse-grip stability ball pulldown	Secondary only	Level 1–4
Pulldown	Sit on a ball	One-hand high-cable pulley	Palm facing in	N/A	One-arm neutral-grip stability ball pulldown	Primary or secondary	Level 1–4
Pulldown	Sit on a ball	One-hand high-cable pulley	Palm facing in	Attach a rope to the pulley	One-arm rope stability ball pulldown	Primary or secondary	Level 1–4
Pulldown	Sit on a ball	Resistance bands	Normal	N/A	Stretch cord stability ball pulldown	Primary or secondary	Level 1–4
Pulldown	Sit on a ball	Resistance bands	Reverse	N/A	Reverse-grip stretch cord stability ball pulldown	Secondary only	Level 1–4
Pulldown	Sit on a ball	Resistance bands	Reverse close-grip	N/A	Close-grip stretch cord stability ball pulldown	Primary or secondary	Level 1–4
Pulldown	Sit on a ball	Resistance bands	Palms facing each other	N/A	Neutral-grip stretch cord stability ball pulldown	Primary or secondary	Level 1–4

The Lucky Thirteen Move	Posture Spin-Off	Tool Spin-Off	Grip Spin-Off	Here's a Twist	Here's What You've Just Created	Here's What Type of Exercise It Is	Who Should Do It?
Pulldown	Stand	Two-hand high-cable pulley	Normal	N/A	Standing pulldown	Primary or secondary	Level 1–4
Pulldown	Stand	Two-hand high-cable pulley	Wide	N/A	Standing wide-grip pulldown	Primary or secondary	Level 1–4
Pulldown	Stand	Two-hand high-cable pulley	Reverse	N/A	Standing reverse-grip pulldown	Secondary only	Level 1–4
Pulldown	Stand	Two-hand high-cable pulley	Reverse close grip	N/A	Standing reverse close-grip pulldown	Primary or secondary	Level 1–4
Pulldown	Stand	Two-hand high-cable pulley	Palms facing each other	N/A	Standing neutral-grip pulldown	Primary or secondary	Level 1–4
Pulldown	Stand	Two-hand high-cable pulley	Palms facing each other	Attach a rope to the pulley	Standing rope pulldown	Primary or secondary	Level 1–4
Pulldown	Stand	One-hand high-cable pulley	Normal	N/A	Standing one-arm pulldown	Primary or secondary	Level 1–4
Pulldown	Stand	One-hand high-cable pulley	Reverse	N/A	Standing one-arm reverse-grip pulldown	Secondary only	Level 1–4
Pulldown	Stand	One-hand high-cable pulley	Palm facing in	N/A	Standing one-arm neutral-grip pulldown	Primary or secondary	Level 1–4
Pulldown	Stand	One-hand high-cable pulley	Palm facing in	Attach a rope to the pulley	Standing one-arm rope pulldown	Primary or secondary	Level 1–4
Pulldown	Stand	Resistance bands	Normal	N/A	Standing stretch cord pulldown	Primary or secondary	Level 1–4
Pulldown	Stand	Resistance bands	Reverse	N/A	Standing reverse-grip stretch cord pulldown	Secondary only	Level 1–4
Pulldown	Stand	Resistance bands	Reverse close grip	N/A	Standing close-grip stretch cord pulldown	Primary or secondary	Level 1–4
Pulldown	Stand	Resistance bands	Palms facing each other	N/A	Standing neutral-grip stretch cord pulldown	Primary or secondary	Level 1–4

KNEELING

The Lucky Thirteen Move	Posture Spin-Off	Tool Spin-Off	Grip Spin-Off	Here's a Twist	Here's What You've Just Created	Here's What Type of Exercise It Is	Who Should Do It?
Pulldown	Kneeling	Two-hand high-cable pulley	Normal	N/A	Kneeling pulldown	Primary or secondary	Level 1–4
Pulldown	Kneeling	Two-hand high-cable pulley	Wide	N/A	Kneeling wide-grip pulldown	Primary or secondary	Level 1–4
Pulldown	Kneeling	Two-hand high-cable pulley	Reverse	N/A	Kneeling reverse-grip pulldown	Secondary only	Level 1–4
Pulldown	Kneeling	Two-hand high-cable pulley	Reverse close grip	N/A	Kneeling reverse close-grip pulldown	Primary or secondary	Level 1–4
Pulldown	Kneeling	Two-hand high-cable pulley	Palms facing each other	N/A	Kneeling neutral-grip pulldown	Primary or secondary	Level 1–4
Pulldown	Kneeling	Two-hand high-cable pulley	Palms facing each other	Attach a rope to the pulley	Kneeling rope pulldown	Primary or secondary	Level 1–4
Pulldown	Kneeling	One-hand high-cable pulley	Normal	N/A	Kneeling one-arm pulldown	Primary or secondary	Level 1–4
Pulldown	Kneeling	One-hand high-cable pulley	Reverse	N/A	Kneeling one-arm reverse-grip pulldown	Secondary only	Level 1–4
Pulldown	Kneeling	One-hand high-cable pulley	Palm facing in	N/A	Kneeling one-arm neutral-grip pulldown	Primary or secondary	Level 1–4
Pulldown	Kneeling	One-hand high-cable pulley	Palm facing in	Attach a rope to the pulley	Kneeling one-arm rope pulldown	Primary or secondary	Level 1–4
Pulldown	Kneeling	Resistance bands	Normal	N/A	Kneeling stretch cord pulldown	Primary or secondary	Level 1–4
Pulldown	Kneeling	Resistance bands	Reverse	N/A	Kneeling reverse-grip stretch cord pulldown	Secondary only	Level 1–4
Pulldown	Kneeling	Resistance bands	Reverse close-grip	N/A	Kneeling close-grip stretch cord pulldown	Primary or secondary	Level 1–4
Pulldown	Kneeling	Resistance bands	Palms facing each other	N/A	Kneeling neutral-grip stretch cord pulldown	Primary or secondary	Level 1–4

HANGING FROM A CHIN-UP BAR

The Lucky Thirteen Move	Posture Spin-Off	Tool Spin-Off	Grip Spin-Off	Here's a Twist	Here's What You've Just Created	Here's What Type of Exercise It Is	Who Should Do It?
Pulldown	Hanging from a bar	None	Normal	N/A	Pull-up	Primary or secondary	Level 1–4
Pulldown	Hanging from a bar	None	Wide	N/A	Wide-grip pull-up	Primary or secondary	Level 1–4
Pulldown	Hanging from a bar	None	Reverse close grip	N/A	Reverse close-grip pull-up	Primary or secondary	Level 1–4
Pulldown	Hanging from a bar	None	Reverse	N/A	Reverse-grip pull-up	Secondary only	Level 1–4
Pulldown	Hanging from a bar	None	Palms facing each other	N/A	Neutral-grip pull-up	Primary or secondary	Level 1–4

6. SPIN-OFF OF THE ROW

SPIN-OFF 1: CHANGE YOUR POSTURE

The Lucky Thirteen Posture: Standing (Bent Over)

Posture Spin-Off 1: Leaning on a Bench

Stand with your left side next to a weight bench with a weight in your right hand. Rest your left hand and knee along the length of the bench and bend forward until your back is almost parallel to the floor. Your right arm should hang straight down, palm neutral. This is the start of the move. Slowly pull the weight straight up to the side of your chest. Keep the "rowing arm elbow" close to your body. Lower the weight back down, repeat until the set is over, then switch positions to work your left side.

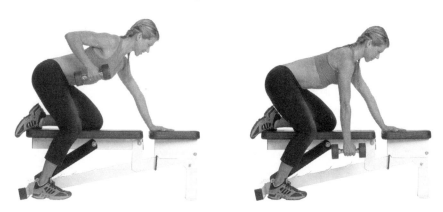

Posture Spin-Off 2: Standing Upright

Stand facing a pulley station, grab the handles, then step back until your arms are fully extended in front of you. This is the start of the move. Slowly pull your elbows straight back as far as possible, keeping your arms close to your sides, then return to the starting position.

Posture Spin-Off 3: Sitting on a Bench

Sit on the edge of a bench facing a pulley station with your feet flat on the floor. Lean forward, grab the handle, then lean back until you are sitting upright with your arms fully extended in front of you. This is the start of the move. Slowly pull your elbows straight back as far as possible, keeping your arms close to your sides, then return to the starting position.

Posture Spin-Off 4: Seated at a Rowing Machine

Sit at a rowing station and place your feet up on the footrests in front of you. Lean forward, grab the handles, then lean back until you are sitting upright with your arms fully extended in front of you. This is the start of the move. Slowly pull your elbows straight back as far as possible, keeping your arms close to your sides, then return to the starting position.

Posture Spin-Off 5: Sitting on a Stability Ball

The same positioning you would use to sit on a bench applies for this posture spin-off as well, only you'll sit on top of a stability ball instead. Sit on a stability ball facing a pulley station with your feet flat on the floor.

SPIN-OFF 2: CHANGE YOUR TOOLS

The Lucky Thirteen Tool: Two Dumbbells

Tool Spin-Off 1: Barbell

Tool Spin-Off 2: One Dumbbell

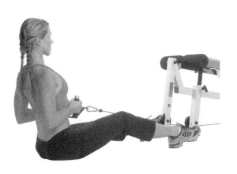

Tool Spin-Off 3: One-Hand
Low- or High-Cable Pulley

For this spin-off, you'll be using a single-cable handle, unless I give you a twist.

Tool Spin-Off 4: Two-Hand Low-
or High-Cable Pulley

For this spin-off, you'll be using a lat pulldown bar attachment, unless I give you a twist.

For this spin-off, attach one end of the resistance band to something sturdy in front of you (or step on one end if you're doing the row from a bent-over posture) and grab the other end in your hand. For any exercises that require you to use resistance bands, you should have an end in each hand to work both arms at the same time.

SPIN-OFF 3: CHANGE YOUR GRIP

The Lucky Thirteen Grip: Normal Grip

Grip Spin-Off 1: Wide Grip (Overhand Grip, Hands Wider Than Shoulder-Width Apart)

Grip Spin-Off 2: Close Grip (Overhand Grip, Hands Closer Than Shoulder-Width Apart)

Grip Spin-Off 3: Reverse Grip (Underhand Grip, Palms Will Either Face Forward or Up, Depending on Your Posture)

Grip Spin-Off 4: Reverse Close Grip (Underhand Grip, Hands Closer Than Shoulder-Width Apart)

Grip Spin-Off 5: Palms Facing Each Other

You'll see this spin-off attached to many of the dumbbell and cable pulley exercises. Just rotate your wrists inward until your palms face toward each other. As you row, keep your wrists in that position so when your hands reach your sides, your palms should still be facing each other.

The Twists to Expect

Twist wrists outward

If your palms face down (or backward, depending on your posture) as you start rowing, you'll twist your wrists outward ninety degrees so that your palms end up facing in toward each other once you've pulled the weight, handle, etc. into your body.

Twist wrists inward

If your palms face up (or forward, depending on your posture) as you start rowing, you'll twist your wrists inward ninety degrees so that your palms end up facing in toward each other once you've pulled the weight, handle, etc. into your body.

Twist wrists inward or outward

If your palms are facing each other as you start rowing, you can twist your wrists inward or outward ninety degrees so that your palms end up facing forward (or up) or backward (or down) once you've pulled the weight into your body.

Attach a rope to the pulley

Using a rope lets you angle your hands in a way that makes the exercise feel different to your back muscles. Just grab the rope with your palms facing in.

READY TO TAKE CHARGE OF YOUR WORKOUTS?

Thought you knew only a handful of exercises to work your back, biceps, and shoulders? Look at what you can do now!

STANDING (BENT OVER AT THE WAIST)

The Lucky Thirteen Move	Posture Spin-Off	Tool Spin-Off	Grip Spin-Off	Here's a Twist	Here's What You've Just Created	Here's What Type of Exercise It Is	Who Should Do It?
The row	Standing (bent over)	Barbell	Normal	N/A	Barbell row	Primary or secondary	Level 1–4
The row	Standing (bent over)	Barbell	Reverse	N/A	Supinated barbell row	Primary or secondary	Level 1–4
The row	Standing (bent over)	Two Dumbbells	Normal	N/A	Dumbbell row	Primary or secondary	Level 1–4
The row	Standing (bent over)	Two Dumbbells	Reverse	N/A	Supinated dumbbell row	Primary or secondary	Level 1–4
The row	Standing (bent over)	Two Dumbbells	Palms facing each other	N/A	Neutral-grip dumbbell row	Primary or secondary	Level 1–4
The row	Standing (bent over)	Two Dumbbells	Normal	Twist wrists outward	Twisting dumbbell row 1	Primary or secondary	Level 2–4
The row	Standing (bent over)	Two Dumbbells	Reverse	Twist wrists inward	Twisting dumbbell row 2	Primary or secondary	Level 2–4
The row	Standing (bent over)	Two Dumbbells	Palms facing each other	Twist wrists inward or outward	Twisting dumbbell row 3	Primary or secondary	Level 2–4
The row	Standing (bent over)	Resistance bands	Palms facing each other	N/A	Neutral-grip stretch cord row	Primary or secondary	Level 1–4

The Lucky Thirteen Move	Posture Spin-Off	Tool Spin-Off	Grip Spin-Off	Here's a Twist	Here's What You've Just Created	Here's What Type of Exercise It Is	Who Should Do It?
The row	Leaning on a bench	One dumbbell	Normal	N/A	One-arm bent-over row	Primary or secondary	Level 1–4
The row	Leaning on a bench	One dumbbell	Reverse	N/A	One-arm reverse-grip bent-over row	Primary or secondary	Level 1–4
The row	Leaning on a bench	One dumbbell	Palm facing in	N/A	One arm neutral-grip bent-over row	Primary or secondary	Level 1–4
The row	Leaning on a bench	One dumbbell	Normal	Twist wrist outward	One-arm bent-over twisting row 1	Primary or secondary	Level 1–4
The row	Leaning on a bench	One dumbbell	Reverse	Twist wrist inward	One-arm bent-over twisting row 2	Primary or secondary	Level 1–4
The row	Leaning on a bench	One dumbbell	Palm facing in	Twist wrist inward or outward	One-arm bent-over twisting row 3	Primary or secondary	Level 1–4
The row	Leaning on a bench	Resistence bands	Palm facing in	N/A	Neutral-grip bent-over stretch cord row	Primary or secondary	Level 1–4

STANDING

The Lucky Thirteen Move	Posture Spin-Off	Tool Spin-Off	Grip Spin-Off	Here's a Twist	Here's What You've Just Created	Here's What Type of Exercise It Is	Who Should Do It?
The row	Stand	One-hand high-cable pulley	Normal	N/A	Standing one-arm cable row	Primary or secondary	Level 1–4
The row	Stand	One-hand high-cable pulley	Reverse	N/A	Standing reverse-grip cable row	Primary or secondary	Level 1–4
The row	Stand	One-hand high-cable pulley	Palm facing in	N/A	Standing neutral-grip cable row	Primary or secondary	Level 1–4
The row	Stand	One-hand high-cable pulley	Normal	Twist wrist outward	Standing twisting cable row 1	Primary or secondary	Level 1–4
The row	Stand	One-hand high-cable pulley	Reverse	Twist wrist inward	Standing twisting cable row 2	Primary or secondary	Level 1–4
The row	Stand	One-hand high-cable pulley	Palm facing in	Twist wrist inward or outward	Standing twisting cable row 3	Primary or secondary	Level 1–4
The row	Stand	Two-hand high-cable pulley	Normal	N/A	Standing two-arm cable row	Primary or secondary	Level 1–4
The row	Stand	Two-hand high-cable pulley	Reverse	N/A	Standing reverse-grip two-arm cable row	Primary or secondary	Level 1–4
The row	Stand	Two-hand high-cable pulley	Palms facing each other	N/A	Standing neutral-grip cable row	Primary or secondary	Level 1–4
The row	Stand	Resistance bands	Palms facing each other	N/A	Standing stretch cord row	Primary or secondary	Level 1–4

The Lucky Thirteen Move	Posture Spin-Off	Tool Spin-Off	Grip Spin-Off	Here's a Twist	Here's What You've Just Created	Here's What Type of Exercise It Is	Who Should Do It?
The row	Sit on a bench (leaning over)	One-hand low-cable pulley	Normal	N/A	Seated one-arm cable row	Primary or secondary	Level 1–4
The row	Sit on a bench (leaning over)	One-hand low-cable pulley	Reverse	N/A	Seated reverse-grip cable row	Primary or secondary	Level 1–4
The row	Sit on a bench (leaning over)	One-hand low-cable pulley	Palm facing in	N/A	Seated neutral-grip cable row	Primary or secondary	Level 1–4
The row	Sit on a bench (leaning over)	One-hand low-cable pulley	Normal	Twist wrist outward	Seated twisting cable row 1	Primary or secondary	Level 1–4
The row	Sit on a bench (leaning over)	One-hand low-cable pulley	Reverse	Twist wrist inward	Seated twisting cable row 2	Primary or secondary	Level 1–4
The row	Sit on a bench (leaning over)	One-hand low-cable pulley	Palm facing in	Twist wrist inward or outward	Seated twisting cable row 3	Primary or secondary	Level 1–4
The row	Sit on a bench (leaning over)	Two-hand low-cable pulley	Normal	N/A	Seated two-arm cable row	Primary or secondary	Level 1–4
The row	Sit on a bench (leaning over)	Two-hand low-cable pulley	Reverse	N/A	Seated reverse-grip two-arm cable row	Primary or secondary	Level 1–4
The row	Sit on a bench (leaning over)	Two-hand low-cable pulley	Palms facing each other	N/A	Seated neutral-grip cable row	Primary or secondary	Level 1–4

SITTING ON A STABILITY BALL

The Lucky Thirteen Move	Posture Spin-Off	Tool Spin-Off	Grip Spin-Off	Here's a Twist	Here's What You've Just Created	Here's What Type of Exercise It Is	Who Should Do It?
The row	Sit on a ball (leaning over)	One-hand low-cable pulley	Normal	N/A	Stability ball one-arm cable row	Primary or secondary	Level 2–4
The row	Sit on a ball (leaning over)	One-hand low-cable pulley	Reverse	N/A	Stability ball reverse-grip cable row	Primary or secondary	Level 2–4
The row	Sit on a ball (leaning over)	One-hand low-cable pulley	Palm facing in	N/A	Stability ball neutral-grip cable row	Primary or secondary	Level 2–4
The row	Sit on a ball (leaning over)	One-hand low-cable pulley	Normal	Twist wrist outward	Stability ball twisting cable row 1	Primary or secondary	Level 2–4
The row	Sit on a ball (leaning over)	One-hand low-cable pulley	Reverse	Twist wrist inward	Stability ball twisting cable row 2	Primary or secondary	Level 2–4
The row	Sit on a ball (leaning over)	One-hand low-cable pulley	Palm facing in	Twist wrist inward or outward	Stability ball twisting cable row 3	Primary or secondary	Level 2–4
The row	Sit on a ball (leaning over)	Two-hand low-cable pulley	Normal	N/A	Stability ball two-arm cable row	Primary or secondary	Level 2–4
The row	Sit on a ball (leaning over)	Two-hand low-cable pulley	Reverse	N/A	Stability ball reverse-grip two-arm cable row	Primary or secondary	Level 2–4
The row	Sit on a ball (leaning over)	Two-hand low-cable pulley	Palms facing each other	N/A	Stability ball neutral-grip cable row	Primary or secondary	Level 2–4
The row	Sit on a ball (leaning over)	Resistance bands	Palms facing each other	N/A	Stability ball stretch cord row	Primary or secondary	Level 2–4

7. SPIN-OFF OF THE SHOULDER PRESS

SPIN-OFF 1: CHANGE YOUR POSTURE

The Lucky Thirteen Posture: Standing

Posture Spin-Off 1: Sitting on a Bench
Sit on the end of a weight bench with your feet flat on the floor. Holding your weights bring your hands up to the outsides of your shoulders, palms facing forward. Your hands should be wider than shoulder-width apart with your elbows pointing down toward the floor.

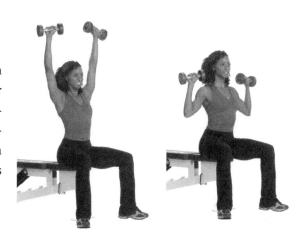

**Posture Spin-Off 2:
Sitting on a Stability Ball**
Sit on top of a stability ball with your legs bent, feet flat on the floor. Holding whichever tool you're using, bring your hands up to the outsides of your shoulders, palms facing forward. Your hands should be wider than shoulder-width apart with your elbows pointing down toward the floor. Once you have your balance, do the move looking forward, keeping your head and back upright as you go.

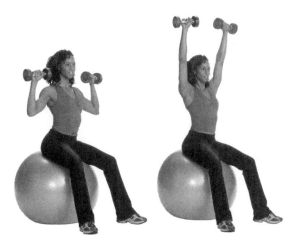

The Lucky Thirteen Tool: Two Dumbbells

Tool Spin-Off 1: Barbell

When using a barbell, grab the bar with your hands slightly wider than shoulder-width apart. Bring your hands up to the outsides of your shoulders so that the middle of the bar is right above the top of your chest.

Tool Spin-Off 2: One Dumbbell

Whenever an exercise asks you to use only one dumbbell, you'll hold it in one hand and place your other hand over your chest during the exercise. Once you've completed the exercise, switch the weight into your opposite hand and repeat the exercise. This one-arm training is a type of unilateral conditioning that helps improve your sense of balance as you exercise. It also ensures that both sides of your body are worked equally, which means your naturally dominant side can't dominate so easily!

Tool Spin-Off 3: Two-Hand Low-Cable Pulley

For this spin-off, you'll be using a lat pulldown bar attachment, unless I give you a twist. Place whatever you're asked to sit on directly in front of, and as close to, the low pulley to start.

Tool Spin-Off 4: Resistance Bands

Step on one end of the resistance band and hold the other end in your hand to work one side at a time. For any exercises that require you to use resistance bands with two hands, you should have an end in each hand and the center appropriately secured to facilitate the movement.

SPIN-OFF 3: CHANGE YOUR GRIP

The Lucky Thirteen Grip: Wide Grip (Wider Than Shoulder-Width Apart, Palms Facing Forward)

Grip Spin-Off 1: Reverse Wide Grip (Shoulder-Width Apart, Palms Facing in Toward You)

The Twists You Can Expect

Twist wrists as you press

If your palms face out before you start pressing, you'll twist your wrists inward ninety degrees so that your palms end up facing each other when your arms are overhead. If your palms face in toward each other before you start pressing, you'll twist your wrists outward ninety degrees so they end up facing forward. Either "twist" helps to engage more of the muscle fibers within your shoulders to fire. You can also vary the amount you twist. Make sure the twist is controlled and not "snapped."

READY TO TAKE CHARGE OF YOUR WORKOUTS?

Thought you knew only a handful of exercises to work your shoulders? Look at what you can do now!

STANDING

The Lucky Thirteen Move	Posture Spin-Off	Tool Spin-Off	Grip Spin-Off	Here's a Twist	Here's What You've Just Created	Here's What Type of Exercise It Is	Who Should Do It?
Shoulder press	Stand	Barbell	Wide	N/A	Barbell press	Primary or secondary	Level 1–4
Shoulder press	Stand	Barbell	Wide	Lower the bar behind your your head	Behind-the-neck barbell press	Primary or secondary	Level 3–4
Shoulder press	Stand	Two dumbbells	Wide	N/A	Dumbbell press	Primary or secondary	Level 1–4
Shoulder press	Stand	Two dumbbells	Palms facing each other	N/A	Parallel-grip dumbbell press	Primary or secondary	Level 1–4
Shoulder press	Stand	Two dumbbells	Wide	Twist wrists as you press	Twisting press 1	Primary or secondary	Level 1–4
Shoulder press	Stand	Two dumbbells	Palms facing each other	Twist wrists as you press	Twisting press 2	Primary or secondary	Level 1–4
Shoulder press	Stand	Two dumbbells	Reverse	Twist wrists 180° as you press	Arnold press *	Primary or secondary	Level 2–4
Shoulder press	Stand	One dumbbell	Wide	N/A	One-arm dumbbell press	Secondary only	Level 3–4
Shoulder press	Stand	One dumbbell	Palm facing in	N/A	One-arm parallel-grip dumbbell press	Secondary only	Level 3–4
Shoulder press	Stand	One dumbbell	Wide	Twist wrist as you press	One-arm twisting press 1	Secondary only	Level 3–4
Shoulder press	Stand	One dumbbell	Palm facing in	Twist wrist as you press	One-arm twisting press 2	Primary or secondary	Level 1–4

The Lucky Thirteen Move	Posture Spin-Off	Tool Spin-Off	Grip Spin-Off	Here's a Twist	Here's What You've Just Created	Here's What Type of Exercise It Is	Who Should Do It?
Shoulder press	Stand	One dumbbell	Reverse	Twist wrist 180° as you press	One-arm Arnold press	Secondary only	Level 3–4
Shoulder press	Stand	Resistance bands	Wide	N/A	Stretch cord press	Primary or secondary	Level 1–4
Shoulder press	Stand	Resistance bands	Palms facing each other	N/A	Stretch cord parallel-grip press	Primary or secondary	Level 1–4
Shoulder press	Stand	Resistance bands	Wide	Twist wrists as you press	Stretch cord twisting press	Primary or secondary	Level 1–4

(*Named after the Governator because he did it first.)

SITTING ON A BENCH

The Lucky Thirteen Move	Posture Spin-Off	Tool Spin-Off	Grip Spin-Off	Here's a Twist	Here's What You've Just Created	Here's What Type of Exercise It Is	Who Should Do It?
Shoulder press	Sit on a bench	Barbell	Wide	N/A	Seated press	Primary or secondary	Level 1–4
Shoulder press	Sit on a bench	Two dumbbells	Wide	N/A	Seated dumbbell press	Primary or secondary	Level 1–4
Shoulder press	Sit on a bench	Two dumbbells	Palms facing each other	N/A	Seated parallel-grip dumbbell press	Primary or secondary	Level 1–4
Shoulder press	Sit on a bench	Two dumbbells	Wide	Twist wrists as you press	Seated twisting press 1	Secondary only	Level 1–4
Shoulder press	Sit on a bench	Two dumbbells	Palms facing each other	Twist wrists as you press	Seated twisting press 2	Primary or secondary	Level 1–4
Shoulder press	Sit on a bench	Two dumbbells	Reverse	Twist wrists 180° as you press	Seated Arnold press	Primary or secondary	Level 2–4
Shoulder press	Sit on a bench	One dumbbell	Wide	N/A	Seated one-arm dumbbell press	Secondary only	Level 3–4
Shoulder press	Sit on a bench	One dumbbell	Palm facing in	N/A	Seated one-arm parallel-grip dumbbell press	Secondary only	Level 3–4
Shoulder press	Sit on a bench	One dumbbell	Wide	Twist wrist outward as you press	Seated one-arm twisting press 1	Secondary only	Level 3–4
Shoulder press	Sit on a bench	One dumbbell	Palm facing in	Twist wrist inward as you press	Seated one-arm twisting press 2	Primary or secondary	Level 1–4

The Lucky Thirteen Move	Posture Spin-Off	Tool Spin-Off	Grip Spin-Off	Here's a Twist	Here's What You've Just Created	Here's What Type of Exercise It Is	Who Should Do It?
Shoulder press	Sit on a bench	One dumbbell	Reverse	Twist wrist 180° as you press	Seated one-arm Arnold press	Secondary only	Level 3–4
Shoulder press	Sit on a bench	Two-hand low-cable pulley	Wide	N/A	Seated cable press	Primary or secondary	Level 1–4
Shoulder press	Sit on a bench	Resistance bands	Wide	N/A	Seated stretch cord press	Primary or secondary	Level 1–4
Shoulder press	Sit on a bench	Resistance bands	Palms facing each other	N/A	Seated stretch cord parallel-grip press	Primary or secondary	Level 1–4
Shoulder press	Sit on a bench	Resistance bands	Wide	Twist wrists as you press	Seated stretch cord twisting press	Primary or secondary	Level 1–4

SITTING ON A STABILITY BALL

The Lucky Thirteen Move	Posture Spin-Off	Tool Spin-Off	Grip Spin-Off	Here's a Twist	Here's What You've Just Created	Here's What Type of Exercise It Is	Who Should Do It?
Shoulder press	Sit on a ball	Barbell	Wide	N/A	Stability ball press	Primary or secondary	Level 1–4
Shoulder press	Sit on a ball	Two dumbbells	Wide	N/A	Stability ball dumbbell press	Primary or secondary	Level 1–4
Shoulder press	Sit on a ball	Two dumbbells	Palms facing each other	N/A	Stability ball parallel-grip dumbbell press	Primary or secondary	Level 1–4
Shoulder press	Sit on a ball	Two dumbbells	Wide	Twist wrists as you press	Stability ball twisting press 1	Secondary only	Level 1–4
Shoulder press	Sit on a ball	Two dumbbells	Palms facing each other	Twist wrists as you press	Stability ball twisting press 2	Primary or secondary	Level 1–4
Shoulder press	Sit on a ball	Two dumbbells	Reverse	Twist wrists 180° as you press	Stability ball Arnold press	Primary or secondary	Level 2–4
Shoulder press	Sit on a ball	One dumbbell	Wide	N/A	Stability ball one-arm dumbbell press	Secondary only	Level 3–4
Shoulder press	Sit on a ball	One dumbbell	Palm facing in	N/A	Stability ball one-arm parallel-grip dumbbell press	Secondary only	Level 3–4
Shoulder press	Sit on a ball	One dumbbell	Wide	Twist wrist outward as you press	Stability ball one-arm twisting press 1	Secondary only	Level 3–4
Shoulder press	Sit on a ball	One dumbbell	Palm facing in	Twist wrist inward as you press	Stability ball one-arm twisting press 2	Primary or secondary	Level 1–4

The Lucky Thirteen Move	Posture Spin-Off	Tool Spin-Off	Grip Spin-Off	Here's a Twist	Here's What You've Just Created	Here's What Type of Exercise It Is	Who Should Do It?
Shoulder press	Sit on a ball	One dumbbell	Reverse	Twist wrist 180° as you press	Stability ball one-arm Arnold press	Secondary only	Level 3–4
Shoulder press	Sit on a ball	Two-hand low-cable pulley	Wide	N/A	Stability ball cable press	Primary or secondary	Level 1–4
Shoulder press	Sit on a ball	Resistance bands	Wide	N/A	Stability ball stretch cord press	Primary or secondary	Level 1–4
Shoulder press	Sit on a ball	Resistance bands	Palms facing each other	N/A	Stability ball stretch cord parallel-grip press	Primary or secondary	Level 1–4
Shoulder press	Sit on a ball	Resistance bands	Wide	Twist wrists as you press	Stability ball stretch cord twisting press	Primary or secondary	Level 1–4

8. SPIN-OFF OF THE RAISE

SPIN-OFF 1: CHANGE YOUR POSTURE

The Lucky Thirteen Posture: Standing

Posture Spin-Off 1: Sitting on a Bench

Sit on a bench with your arms at your sides and a light dumbbell in each hand, palms facing each other. Keeping your arms straight, slowly raise them out to your sides until they're parallel to the floor (you'll look like the letter "T"). Slowly lower your arms back down to your sides.

Posture Spin-Off 2: Sitting on a Stability Ball

Sit on a stability ball with your arms at your sides and a light dumbbell in each hand, palms facing each other. Keeping your arms straight, slowly raise them out to your sides until they're parallel to the floor. Slowly lower your arms back down to your sides.

Posture Spin-Off 3: Bent Over

With a dumbbell in each hand, bend forward at the waist until your back is almost parallel to the floor. Your legs should be straight (knees unlocked) with your arms hanging straight down, palms facing each other. Slowly raise the dumbbells out to each side until your arms are parallel to the floor, then lower your arms back down.

GUNNAR'S TIP

If you have a hard time maintaining your balance with this posture, try sitting on a bench and leaning forward until your chest reaches your knees instead. Work your way up to standing.

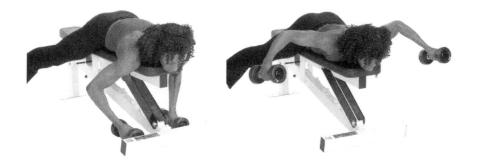

Posture Spin-Off 4: Lying Facedown on a Bench

Lie facedown on a flat bench with a light dumbbell in each hand, letting your arms hang straight down to the floor, palms facing each other. If your arms are too long (or the bench is too short), you can also lie facedown on an incline bench instead. Keeping your arms straight (elbows unlocked), slowly raise them out from your sides until they're parallel to the floor, then lower them back down. I would advise putting a towel on the bench for a multitude of reasons, but that's just me.

SPIN-OFF 2: CHANGE YOUR TOOLS

The Lucky Thirteen Tool: Two Dumbbells

Tool Spin-Off 1: Two-Hand Low-Cable Pulley

This spin-off will require a cable crossover machine with two low pulley stations. Stand between the two cable towers with your feet about shoulder-width apart. Cross your hands in front of you, lean down and grab a pulley in each hand. Your left hand will be holding the right cable pulley and your right hand will be holding the left cable pulley. Your arms should be hanging below you with your hands crossed over each other. This is the start of the move. With your elbows bent, slowly raise your arms out to your sides until they are parallel to the floor, then slowly lower your arms back down, and repeat.

Tool Spin-Off 2: One-Hand Low-Cable Pulley

To do this spin-off, get in the same position that you would when using the two-hand low-cable pulley. Instead of grabbing both handles, grab just one and work each arm individually. You can place your nonworking hand either on the small of your back or your abs or let your arm hang straight down. Placing it on the hip is fine as well; I just think it looks very '80s. . . .

Tool Spin-Off 3: Resistance Bands

Use this spin-off tool in the same way you would the one- or two-hand cable pulley. Just tie one end of the cord to a sturdy object on the floor and stand alongside it. Grab the other end with whichever hand is farther away from the object (if the object is on your left side, then reach down and grab the other end with your right hand, and vice versa).

SPIN-OFF 3: CHANGE YOUR GRIP

The Lucky Thirteen Grip: Palms Facing Each Other

Grip Spin-Off 1: Normal Grip (Overhand Grip, Palms Will Either Face Behind You or Down, Depending on Your Posture)

The Twists to Expect

Raise one arm at a time

Instead of lifting both arms up together, lift only your left arm. Once you lower your left arm back down, raise your right arm. Working each arm separately makes it easier to focus on each shoulder, and it also makes it more difficult to use momentum to cheat the weight up.

READY TO TAKE CHARGE OF YOUR WORKOUTS?

Thought you knew only a handful of exercises to work your shoulders (deltoids)? Look at what you can do now!

The Lucky Thirteen Move	Posture Spin-Off	Tool Spin-Off	Grip Spin-Off	Here's a Twist	Here's What You've Just Created	Here's What Type of Exercise It Is	Who Should Do It?
Raise	Stand	Two dumbbells	Palms facing each other	N/A	Side lateral raise 1	Primary or secondary	Level 1–4
Raise	Stand	Two dumbbells	Normal	N/A	Side lateral raise 2	Primary or secondary	Level 1–4
Raise	Stand	Two dumbbells	Palms facing each other or normal	Raise one arm at a time	Single-arm side lateral raise	Primary or secondary	Level 1–4
Raise	Stand	Two-hand low-cable pulley	Palms facing each other	N/A	Two-hand cable side lateral raise 1	Primary or secondary	Level 1–4
Raise	Stand	Two-hand low-cable pulley	Normal	N/A	Two-hand cable side lateral raise 2	Primary or secondary	Level 1–4
Raise	Stand	One-hand low-cable pulley	Palm facing in	N/A	Single-arm cable side lateral raise 1	Primary or secondary	Level 1–4
Raise	Stand	One-hand low-cable pulley	Normal	N/A	Single-arm cable side lateral raise 2	Primary or secondary	Level 1–4
Raise	Stand	Resistance bands	Palms facing each other	N/A	Stretch cord side lateral raise 1	Primary or secondary	Level 1–4
Raise	Stand	Resistance bands	Normal	N/A	Stretch cord side lateral raise 2	Primary or secondary	Level 1–4
Raise	Stand	Resistance bands	Palms facing each other or normal	Raise one arm at a time	Single-arm stretch cord side lateral raise	Primary or secondary	Level 1–4

SITTING ON A BENCH

The Lucky Thirteen Move	Posture Spin-Off	Tool Spin-Off	Grip Spin-Off	Here's a Twist	Here's What You've Just Created	Here's What Type of Exercise It Is	Who Should Do It?
Raise	Sit on a bench	Two dumbbells	Palms facing each other	N/A	Seated side lateral raise 1	Primary or secondary	Level 1–4
Raise	Sit on a bench	Two dumbbells	Normal	N/A	Seated side lateral raise 2	Primary or secondary	Level 1–4
Raise	Sit on a bench	Two dumbbells	Palms facing each other or normal	Raise one arm at a time	Seated single-arm side lateral raise	Primary or secondary	Level 1–4
Raise	Sit on a bench	Resistance bands	Palms facing each other	N/A	Seated stretch cord side lateral raise 1	Primary or secondary	Level 1–4
Raise	Sit on a bench	Resistance bands	Normal	N/A	Seated stretch cord side lateral raise 2	Primary or secondary	Level 1–4
Raise	Sit on a bench	Resistance bands	Palms facing each other or normal	Raise one arm at a time	Seated single-arm stretch cord side lateral raise	Primary or secondary	Level 1–4

SITTING ON A STABILITY BALL

The Lucky Thirteen Move	Posture Spin-Off	Tool Spin-Off	Grip Spin-Off	Here's a Twist	Here's What You've Just Created	Here's What Type of Exercise It Is	Who Should Do It?
Raise	Sit on a ball	Two dumbbells	Palms facing each other	N/A	Stability ball side lateral raise 1	Primary or secondary	Level 2–4
Raise	Sit on a ball	Two dumbbells	Normal	N/A	Stability ball side lateral raise 2	Primary or secondary	Level 2–4
Raise	Sit on a ball	Two dumbbells	Palms facing each other or normal	Raise one arm at a time	Stability ball single-arm side lateral raise	Primary or secondary	Level 2–4
Raise	Sit on a ball	Resistance bands	Palms facing each other	N/A	Stability ball stretch cord side lateral raise 1	Primary or secondary	Level 2–4
Raise	Sit on a ball	Resistance bands	Normal	N/A	Stability ball stretch cord side lateral raise 2	Primary or secondary	Level 2–4
Raise	Sit on a ball	Resistance bands	Palms facing each other or normal	Raise one arm at a time	Stability ball single-arm stretch cord side lateral raise	Primary or secondary	Level 2–4

BENT OVER
(Leaning forward from a standing position)

The Lucky Thirteen Move	Posture Spin-Off	Tool Spin-Off	Grip Spin-Off	Here's a Twist	Here's What You've Just Created	Here's What Type of Exercise It Is	Who Should Do It?
Raise	Bent over	Two dumbbells	Palms facing each other	N/A	Rear lateral raise 1	Secondary only	Level 1–4
Raise	Bent over	Two dumbbells	Normal	N/A	Rear lateral raise 2	Secondary only	Level 1–4
Raise	Bent over	Two dumbbells	Palms facing each other or normal	Raise one arm at a time	Single-arm rear lateral raise	Secondary only	Level 1–4
Raise	Bent over	Two-hand low-cable pulley	Palms facing each other	N/A	Two-hand cable rear lateral raise 1	Secondary only	Level 1–4
Raise	Bent over	Two-hand low-cable pulley	Normal	N/A	Two-hand cable rear lateral raise 2	Secondary only	Level 1–4
Raise	Bent over	One-hand low-cable pulley	Palm facing in	N/A	Single-arm cable rear lateral raise 1	Secondary only	Level 1–4
Raise	Bent over	One-hand low-cable pulley	Normal	N/A	Single-arm cable rear lateral raise 2	Primary or secondary	Level 1–4
Raise	Bent over	Resistance bands	Palms facing each other	N/A	Stretch cord rear lateral raise 1	Secondary only	Level 1–4
Raise	Bent over	Resistance bands	Normal	N/A	Stretch cord rear lateral raise 2	Secondary only	Level 1–4
Raise	Bent over	Resistance bands	Palms facing each other or normal	Raise one arm at a time	Single-arm stretch cord rear lateral raise	Secondary only	Level 1–4

LYING FACEDOWN ON A BENCH

The Lucky Thirteen Move	Posture Spin-Off	Tool Spin-Off	Grip Spin-Off	Here's a Twist	Here's What You've Just Created	Here's What Type of Exercise It Is	Who Should Do It?
Raise	Lie facedown on a bench	Two dumbbells	Palms facing each other	N/A	Lying rear lateral raise 1	Secondary only	Level 1–4
Raise	Lie facedown on a bench	Two dumbbells	Normal	N/A	Lying rear lateral raise 2	Secondary only	Level 1–4
Raise	Lie facedown on a bench	Two dumbbells	Palms facing each other or normal	Raise one arm at a time	Lying single-arm rear lateral raise	Secondary only	Level 1–4
Raise	Lie facedown on a bench	Resistance bands	Palms facing each other	N/A	Lying stretch cord rear lateral raise 1	Secondary only	Level 1–4
Raise	Lie facedown on a bench	Resistance bands	Normal	N/A	Lying stretch cord rear lateral raise 2	Secondary only	Level 1–4
Raise	Lie facedown on a bench	Resistance bands	Palms facing each other or normal	Raise one arm at a time	Lying single-arm stretch cord rear lateral raise	Secondary only	Level 1–4

9. SPIN-OFF OF THE PRESSDOWN

SPIN-OFF 1: CHANGE YOUR TOOLS

The Lucky Thirteen Tool: Two-Hand High-Cable Pulley

Tool Spin-Off 1: One-Hand High-Cable Pulley
For this spin-off, you'll be using a single-cable handle, unless I give you a twist.

Tool Spin-Off 2: Resistance Bands
For this spin-off, you can loop the middle of the stretch cord over a chin-up bar, the edge of a door, or anything high enough to let you grab both ends and pull them down with resistance.

SPIN-OFF 2: CHANGE YOUR GRIP

The Lucky Thirteen grip: Close Grip
(Hands Approximately Twelve Inches Apart, Palms Down)

Grip Spin-Off 1: Close-Grip Reverse Grip (Hands Six to Twelve Inches Apart, Palms Up)

Grip Spin-Off 2: Palms Facing Toward Each Other

The Twists to Expect

Attach a rope to the pulley
What happened to the bar? Using a rope allows you to angle your hands in a unique slant that lets you strengthen different muscle fibers within your triceps.

Attach a Tri-V Bar
This V-shaped bar angles your hands in toward each other, alleviating some stress on your wrists.

READY TO TAKE CHARGE OF YOUR WORKOUTS?

Thought you knew only a handful of exercises to work your triceps?
Look at what you can do now!

STANDING

The Lucky Thirteen Move	Posture Spin-Off	Tool Spin-Off	Grip Spin-Off	Here's a Twist	Here's What You've Just Created	Here's What Type of Exercise It Is	Who Should Do It?
Triceps pressdown	Stand	Two-hand high-cable pulley	Normal	N/A	Triceps pressdown	Primary or secondary	Level 1–4
Triceps pressdown	Stand	Two-hand high-cable pulley	Reverse	N/A	Reverse-grip triceps pressdown	Secondary only	Level 2–4
Triceps pressdown	Stand	Two-hand high-cable pulley	Palms facing each other	Attach a rope to the pulley	Rope triceps pressdown	Primary or secondary	Level 1–4
Triceps pressdown	Stand	Two-hand high-cable pulley	Palms facing each other	Attach a Tri-V bar to the pulley	Tri-V bar triceps pressdown	Primary or secondary	Level 1–4
Triceps pressdown	Stand	One-hand high-cable pulley	Normal	N/A	One-arm triceps pressdown	Primary or secondary	Level 1–4
Triceps pressdown	Stand	One-hand high-cable pulley	Reverse	N/A	Reverse-grip one-arm triceps pressdown	Secondary only	Level 1–4
Triceps pressdown	Stand	One-hand high-cable pulley	Palm facing in	Attach a rope to the pulley	One-arm rope triceps pressdown	Primary or secondary	Level 1–4
Triceps pressdown	Stand	Resistance bands	Palms facing each other	N/A	Stretch cord triceps pressdown	Primary or secondary	Level 1–4

10. SPIN-OFF OF THE EXTENSION

SPIN-OFF 1: CHANGE YOUR POSTURE

The Lucky Thirteen Posture: Standing

Posture Spin-Off 1: Sitting on a Bench

Sit on the end of an exercise bench (or a sturdy chair) with your back straight and your feet firmly on the floor. Grab a single dumbbell with both hands and raise the weight above

your head, rotating it so it is vertical and the top plate rests comfortably on the palms of both your hands, thumbs around the handle. This is starting position for the move. Slowly lower the weight behind your head until your forearms are parallel to the floor, then straighten your arms back over your head.

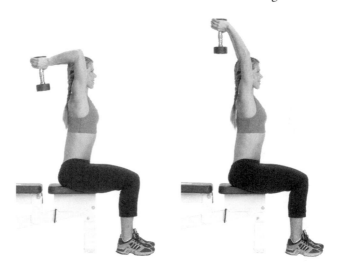

Posture Spin-Off 2: Lying on a Bench

This posture has you extending your arms over your chest instead of your head, but the basic movement is still the same. However, it works only using certain spin-off tools. Lie flat on a bench with your knees bent and feet flat on the floor. Hold a pair of light dumbbells and extend your arms straight up over your chest, palms facing each other. Keeping your upper arms stationary, bend your elbows and slowly lower the weights toward your shoulders.

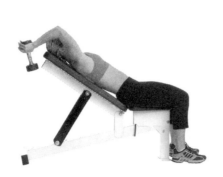 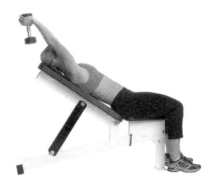

Slowly lift the weights by extending your arms back over your chest. Keep your arms angled slightly back toward your head to keep the triceps engaged throughout the movement.

Posture Spin-Off 3: Sitting on a Stability Ball
Sit on top of a stability ball with your back straight and your feet firmly on the floor. Grab a single dumbbell with both hands and raise the weight above your head, rotating it so it is vertical and the top plate rests comfortably on the palms of both your hands, thumbs around the handle. This is the starting position of the move. Maintaining your balance on the ball, slowly lower the weight behind your head until your forearms are parallel to the floor, then straighten your arms back over your head.

Posture Spin-Off 4: Lying on an Incline Bench
Lie on your back, grab whichever tool you're using, and extend your arms overhead. Even though your upper body is now at an angle, your arms should still be straight above you and perpendicular to the floor. Slowly bend your elbows so that your hands lower down behind the sides of your head. Extend your arms back up until they're straight above you once again.

SPIN-OFF 2: CHANGE YOUR TOOLS

The Lucky Thirteen Tool: One Dumbbell

Tool Spin-Off 1: Two Dumbbells
For this spin-off, you'll hold two lighter dumbbells (one in each hand) with your palms facing in toward each other.

Tool Spin-Off 2: Barbell

This spin-off just substitutes the barbell for the dumbbell. Take a light barbell with your hands closer than shoulder-width apart and extend it overhead the same way you would with a single dumbbell, palms facing forward.

Tool Spin-Off 3: E-Z Curl Bar

Using an E-Z curl bar as a spin-off can make it easier than a barbell if you have problems or discomfort in your wrists. Just grab it with a close grip and extend your arms up above you, palms facing forward.

Tool Spin-Off 4: Two-Hand Low-Cable Pulley

For this spin-off, attach a small straight bar to a low-cable pulley and sit facing away from the weight stack. Reach back, grab the bar, and raise your hands up until your arms are in the same position they would be in after lowering the dumbbell behind your head (arms bent, upper arms in close to your head with your elbows pointing up). Extend your arms overhead, then lower the bar back down behind your head.

Tool Spin-Off 5: Medicine Ball

For this spin-off, raise the ball up, holding it with both hands. Keeping your upper arms close to your ears, slowly bend your elbows to lower the ball behind your head. Extend your arms back overhead. It should feel as though the ball is cocked and ready to be thrown.

Tool Spin-Off 5: Resistance Bands

For this spin-off, you can either tie one end of the cord to a low sturdy object or hold the cord yourself to do each arm individually. To do it, wrap one end of the cord around your right hand and place your hand behind your head so that the length of tubing falls down your back. Reach behind your back with your left hand and grab the other end of the cord so that there isn't any slack. Your right elbow should be pointing upward, your left elbow outward. Next, extend your right arm until it's straight above your head. (You should feel tension coming from the cord; otherwise, you need to grab higher up the cord with your left hand.) Slowly lower your arm back down, repeat for one set, then switch hands to work your other arm.

SPIN-OFF 3: CHANGE YOUR GRIP

The Lucky Thirteen Grip: Close Grip (Overhand Grip; Palms Will Face Forward or Up, Depending on What Tool You're Using)

Grip Spin-Off 1: Palms Facing Each Other

The Twists to Expect

Use one arm

Instead of holding a heavier weight with both hands, grab a lighter weight with your left hand and extend your left arm above you. (Your right hand can cup the elbow of your left arm for support.) Bending only at the elbow, slowly lower the weight down, then raise the weight back up above you by straightening your arm. After your set, switch positions to work your right arm.

Attach a rope to the pulley

Using a rope lets you angle your hands in a unique slant that lets you strengthen different muscle fibers within your triceps.

Attach a Tri-V bar

This V-shaped bar angles your hands in toward each other, alleviating some stress on your wrists.

READY TO TAKE CHARGE OF YOUR WORKOUTS?

Thought you knew only a handful of exercises to work your triceps? Look at what you can do now!

The Lucky Thirteen Move	Posture Spin-Off	Tool Spin-Off	Grip Spin-Off	Here's a Twist	Here's What You've Just Created	Here's What Type of Exercise It Is	Who Should Do It?
Triceps extension	Stand	One dumbbell	Palms facing each other	N/A	Dumbbell triceps extension	Primary or secondary	Level 1–4
Triceps extension	Stand	One dumbbell	Close	Use one-arm at a time	Single-arm dumbbell triceps extension	Primary or secondary	Level 3–4
Triceps extension	Stand	Two dumbbells	Palms facing each other	N/A	Two-arm dumbbell triceps extension	Primary or secondary	Level 1–4
Triceps extension	Stand	Medicine ball	Palms facing each other	N/A	Medicine ball triceps extension	Primary or secondary	Level 1–4
Triceps extension	Stand	E-Z curl bar	Close	N/A	E-Z bar French press	Primary or secondary	Level 3–4
Triceps extension	Stand	Barbell	Close	N/A	French press	Primary or secondary	Level 2–4

SITTING ON A BENCH (OR STURDY CHAIR)

The Lucky Thirteen Move	Posture Spin-Off	Tool Spin-Off	Grip Spin-Off	Here's a Twist	Here's What You've Just Created	Here's What Type of Exercise It Is	Who Should Do It?
Triceps extension	Sit on a bench	One dumbbell	Palms facing each other	N/A	Seated dumbbell triceps extension	Primary or secondary	Level 1–4
Triceps extension	Sit on a bench	One dumbbell	Close	Use one arm at a time	Seated one-arm dumbbell triceps extension	Primary or secondary	Level 3–4
Triceps extension	Sit on a bench	Two dumbbells	Palms facing each other	N/A	Seated two-arm dumbbell triceps extension	Primary or secondary	Level 1–4
Triceps extension	Sit on a bench	Two-hand low-cable pulley	Close	N/A	Seated cable triceps extension 1	Primary or secondary	Level 3–4
Triceps extension	Sit on a bench	Two-hand low-cable pulley	Close	Attach a Tri-V bar	Seated cable triceps extension 2	Primary or secondary	Level 1–4
Triceps extension	Sit on a bench	Two-hand low-cable pulley	Palms facing each other	Attach a rope to the pulley	Seated rope triceps extension	Primary or secondary	Level 1–4
Triceps extension	Sit on a bench	Medicine ball	Palms facing each other	N/A	Seated medicine ball triceps extension	Primary or secondary	Level 1–4
Triceps extension	Sit on a bench	Resistance bands	Palms facing each other	N/A	Seated stretch cord triceps extension	Primary or secondary	Level 1–4
Triceps extension	Sit on a bench	E-Z curl bar	Close	N/A	Seated E-Z bar French press	Primary or secondary	Level 2–4
Triceps extension	Sit on a bench	Barbell	Close	N/A	Seated French press	Primary or secondary	Level 2–4

LYING ON A FLAT BENCH

The Lucky Thirteen Move	Posture Spin-Off	Tool Spin-Off	Grip Spin-Off	Here's a Twist	Here's What You've Just Created	Here's What Type of Exercise It Is	Who Should Do It?
Triceps extension	Lie flat on a bench	One dumbbell	Close	Use one arm at a time	Lying one-arm dumbbell triceps extension	Primary or secondary	Level 3–4
Triceps extension	Lie flat on a bench	Two dumbbells	Palms facing each other	N/A	Lying two-arm dumbbell triceps extension	Primary or secondary	Level 1–4
Triceps extension	Lie flat on a bench	Two-hand low-cable pulley	Close	N/A	Lying cable triceps extension 1	Primary or secondary	Level 3–4
Triceps extension	Lie flat on a bench	Two-hand low-cable pulley	Close	Attach a Tri-V bar	Lying cable triceps extension 2	Primary or secondary	Level 1–4
Triceps extension	Lie flat on a bench	Two-hand low-cable pulley	Palms facing each other	Attach a rope to the pulley	Lying rope triceps extension	Primary or secondary	Level 1–4
Triceps extension	Lie flat on a bench	Medicine ball	Palms facing each other	N/A	Lying medicine ball triceps extension	Primary or secondary	Level 1–4
Triceps extension	Lie flat on a bench	Resistance bands	Palms facing each other	N/A	Lying stretch cord triceps extension	Primary or secondary	Level 1–4
Triceps extension	Lie flat on a bench	E-Z curl bar	Close	N/A	Lying E-Z bar French press	Primary or secondary	Level 2–4
Triceps extension	Lie flat on a bench	Barbell	Close	N/A	Lying French press	Primary or secondary	Level 2–4

SITTING ON A STABILITY BALL

The Lucky Thirteen Move	Posture Spin-Off	Tool Spin-Off	Grip Spin-Off	Here's a Twist	Here's What You've Just Created	Here's What Type of Exercise It Is	Who Should Do It?
Triceps extension	Sit on a ball	One dumbbell	Palms facing each other	N/A	Stability ball dumbbell triceps extension	Primary or secondary	Level 2–4
Triceps extension	Sit on a ball	One dumbbell	Close	Use one arm at a time	Stability ball one-arm dumbbell triceps extension	Primary or secondary	Level 2–4
Triceps extension	Sit on a ball	Two dumbbells	Palms facing each other	N/A	Stability ball two-arm dumbbell triceps extension	Primary or secondary	Level 2–4
Triceps extension	Sit on a ball	Two-hand low-cable pulley	Close	N/A	Stability ball cable triceps extension 1	Primary or secondary	Level 2–4
Triceps extension	Sit on a ball	Two-hand low-cable pulley	Close	Attach a Tri-V bar	Stability ball cable triceps extension 2	Primary or secondary	Level 2–4
Triceps extension	Sit on a ball	Two-hand low-cable pulley	Palms facing each other	Attach a rope to the pulley	Stability ball rope triceps extension	Primary or secondary	Level 2–4
Triceps extension	Sit on a ball	Medicine ball	Palms facing each other	N/A	Stability ball medicine ball triceps extension	Primary or secondary	Level 2–4
Triceps extension	Sit on a ball	Resistance bands	Palms facing each other	N/A	Stability ball stretch cord triceps extension	Primary or secondary	Level 2–4
Triceps extension	Sit on a ball	E-Z curl bar	Close	N/A	Stability ball E-Z bar French press	Primary or secondary	Level 2–4
Triceps extension	Sit on a ball	Barbell	Close	N/A	Stability ball French press	Primary or secondary	Level 2–4

LYING ON AN INCLINE BENCH

The Lucky Thirteen Move	Posture Spin-Off	Tool Spin-Off	Grip Spin-Off	Here's a Twist	Here's What You've Just Created	Here's What Type of Exercise It Is	Who Should Do It?
Triceps extension	Lie on an incline bench	One dumbbell	Close	Use one arm at a time	Incline one-arm dumbbell triceps extension	Primary or secondary	Level 1–4
Triceps extension	Lie on an incline bench	Two dumbbells	Palms facing each other	N/A	Incline two-arm dumbbell triceps extension	Primary or secondary	Level 1–4
Triceps extension	Lie on an incline bench	Two-hand low-cable pulley	Close	N/A	Incline cable triceps extension 1	Primary or secondary	Level 2–4
Triceps extension	Lie on an incline bench	Two-hand low-cable pulley	Close	Attach a Tri-V bar	Incline cable triceps extension 2	Primary or secondary	Level 2–4
Triceps extension	Lie on an incline bench	Two-hand low-cable pulley	Palms facing each other	Attach a rope to the pulley	Incline rope triceps extension	Primary or secondary	Level 2–4
Triceps extension	Lie on an incline bench	Medicine ball	Palms facing each other	N/A	Incline medicine ball triceps extension	Primary or secondary	Level 1–4
Triceps extension	Lie on an incline bench	Resistance bands	Palms facing each other	N/A	Incline stretch cord triceps extension	Primary or secondary	Level 1–4
Triceps extension	Lie on an incline bench	E-Z curl bar	Close	N/A	Incline E-Z bar French press	Primary or secondary	Level 2–4
Triceps extension	Lie on an incline bench	Barbell	Close	N/A	Incline French press	Primary or secondary	Level 2–4

11. SPIN-OFF OF THE CURL

SPIN-OFF 1: CHANGE YOUR POSTURE

The Lucky Thirteen Posture: Standing

Posture Spin-Off 1: Sitting on a Bench

Sit on the edge of a weight bench (or a sturdy chair with no arms along its sides). Your legs should be bent (feet flat on the floor), and your arms should hang straight down from your sides, palms facing forward. While doing the move, keep your head and back straight and look forward, not down at your arms. You can look at your arms later when you're flexing in the mirror. Don't worry, everyone does. . . .

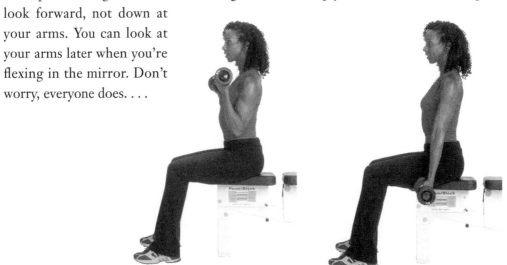

Posture Spin-Off 2: Lying on an Incline Bench

Sit and lie back on the bench with your legs bent, feet flat on the floor. Let your arms hang straight down so that they're perpendicular to the floor (don't worry if they're not in line with your torso—they're not supposed to be). Keep your head and back flat on the bench as you curl the weight up.

Posture Spin-Off 3: Sitting on a Stability Ball

Sit on top of a stability ball with your legs bent, feet flat on the floor. Let your arms hang down straight from your sides, palms facing forward. Once you have your balance, you'll do the move looking forward, keeping your head and back upright as you go.

Posture Spin-Off 4: Sitting at a Preacher Curl Bench

This unique bench lets you isolate your biceps muscles by making it virtually impossible to cheat using momentum. Sit down, place your arms over the padded rest in front of you, and shift yourself forward until you feel the top of the armrest against the middle of your armpits. With your arms straight (palms facing up) and your head facing forward, curl the weight up to the front of your shoulders.
Control the weight throughout the movement; be careful not to hit yourself in the face at the top. It happens. Painful for the person, funny for the trainer.

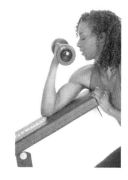

SPIN-OFF 2: CHANGE YOUR TOOLS
The Lucky Thirteen Tool: Two Dumbbells

Tool Spin-Off 1: Barbell

Tool Spin-Off 2: One Dumbbell

Tool Spin-Off 3: One-Hand Low-Cable Pulley
For this spin-off, you'll be using a single-cable handle, unless I give you a twist.

Tool Spin-Off 4. Two-Hand Low-Cable Pulley
For this spin-off, you'll be using a lat pulldown bar attachment, unless I give you a twist.

Tool Spin-Off 5: Resistance Bands

Step on one end of the resistance band and grab the other end in your hand to work one arm at a time. For any exercises that require you to use resistance bands, you should have an end in each hand to work both arms at the same time.

Tool Spin-Off 6: E-Z Curl Bar

SPIN-OFF 3: CHANGE YOUR GRIP

The Lucky Thirteen Grip: Normal Grip

Grip Spin-Off 1: Wide Grip (Palms Forward)

Grip Spin-Off 2: Close Grip (Palms Forward)

Grip Spin-Off 3: Reverse Grip (Palms Down)

Rotate your wrists inward so that the back of your hands face forward in the down position. Your palms should be facing behind you at the start of the movement.

Grip Spin-Off 4: Reverse Wide Grip (Palms Down)

Grip Spin-Off 5: Reverse Close Grip (Palms Down)

Grip Spin-Off 6: Palms Facing Each Other

You'll see this spin-off attached to many of the dumbbell and resistance band exercises. Just rotate your wrists inward until your palms face in toward your thighs. As you curl, keep your wrists in that position so when your hands reach your shoulders at the top, your palms should still be facing each other.

The Twists to Expect

Twist wrists as you curl

If your palms face each other before you start curling, you'll twist your wrists outward ninety degrees so that your palms end up facing in toward your shoulders. This twist helps engage more of the muscle fibers within your forearms.

Stand flat against a wall

Pressing yourself flat against a wall makes cheating impossible, since you can't lean back as you curl to help raise the weight.

What happened to the bar? Actually, using a rope lets you position your hands at a different angle that feels entirely new to your biceps muscles.

READY TO TAKE CHARGE OF YOUR WORKOUTS?

Thought you knew only a handful of exercises to work your biceps? Look at what you can do now!

STANDING

The Lucky Thirteen Move	Posture Spin-Off	Tool Spin-Off	Grip Spin-Off	Here's a Twist	Here's What You've Just Created	Here's What Type of Exercise It Is	Who Should Do It?
Biceps curl	Stand	Barbell	Normal	N/A	Barbell curl	Primary or secondary	Level 1—4
Biceps curl	Stand	Barbell	Wide	N/A	Wide-grip barbell curl	Primary or secondary	Level 3—4
Biceps curl	Stand	Barbell	Close	N/A	Close-grip barbell curl	Primary or secondary	Level 3—4
Biceps curl	Stand	Barbell	Reverse	N/A	Reverse-grip barbell curl	Secondary only	Level 2—4
Biceps curl	Stand	Barbell	Normal, wide, close or reverse	Stand flat along a wall	Wall barbell curl	Primary or secondary	Level 2—4
Biceps curl	Stand	Two dumbells	Normal	N/A	Dumbbell curl	Primary or secondary	Level 1—4
Biceps curl	Stand	Two dumbells	Reverse	N/A	Reverse-grip dumbbell curl	Secondary only	Level 2—4
Biceps curl	Stand	Two dumbells	Palms facing each other	N/A	Hammer curl	Primary or secondary	Level 1—4
Biceps curl	Stand	Two dumbells	Palms facing each other	Twist wrists as you curl	Twisting dumbbell curl	Primary or secondary	Level 1—4
Biceps curl	Stand	Two dumbells	Normal or reverse	Stand flat along a wall	Wall dumbbell curl	Primary or secondary	Level 1—4
Biceps curl	Stand	One-hand low-cable pulley	Normal	N/A	One-arm cable curl	Primary or secondary	Level 1—4
Biceps curl	Stand	One-hand low-cable pulley	Reverse	N/A	One-arm reverse cable curl	Secondary only	Level 2—4
Biceps curl	Stand	One-hand low-cable pulley	Palm facing in	Attach a rope to the pulley	One-arm rope curl	Secondary only	Level 2—4

The Lucky Thirteen Move	Posture Spin-Off	Tool Spin-Off	Grip Spin-Off	Here's a Twist	Here's What You've Just Created	Here's What Type of Exercise It Is	Who Should Do It?
Biceps curl	Stand	Two-hand low-cable pulley	Normal	N/A	Two-hand cable curl	Primary or secondary	Level 1–4
Biceps curl	Stand	Two-hand low-cable pulley	Wide	N/A	Two-hand wide-grip cable curl	Secondary only	Level 3–4
Biceps curl	Stand	Two-hand low-cable pulley	Close	N/A	Two-hand close-grip cable curl	Primary or secondary	Level 3–4
Biceps curl	Stand	Two-hand low-cable pulley	Reverse close grip	N/A	Two-hand reverse-grip cable curl	Secondary only	Level 1–4
Biceps curl	Stand	Two-hand low-cable pulley	Palms facing each other	Attach a rope to the pulley	Two-hand rope curl	Secondary only	Level 1–4
Biceps curl	Stand	Resistance bands	Normal	N/A	Stretch cord curl	Primary or secondary	Level 1–4
Biceps curl	Stand	Resistance bands	Reverse	N/A	Stretch cord reverse curl	Secondary only	Level 1–4
Biceps curl	Stand	Resistance bands	Palms facing each other	N/A	Stretch cord hammer curl	Primary or secondary	Level 1–4
Biceps curl	Stand	E-Z curl bar	Normal	N/A	E-Z bar curl	Primary or secondary	Level 1–4
Biceps curl	Stand	E-Z curl bar	Wide	N/A	Wide-grip E-Z bar curl	Primary or secondary	Level 3–4
Biceps curl	Stand	E-Z curl bar	Close	N/A	Close-grip E-Z bar curl	Primary or secondary	Level 2–4
Biceps curl	Stand	E-Z curl bar	Reverse	N/A	Reverse-grip E-Z bar curl	Secondary only	Level 1–4

SITTING ON A BENCH

The Lucky Thirteen Move	Posture Spin-Off	Tool Spin-Off	Grip Spin-Off	Here's a Twist	Here's What You've Just Created	Here's What Type of Exercise It Is	Who Should Do It?
Biceps curl	Sit on a bench	Two dumbbells	Normal	N/A	Seated dumbbell curl	Primary or secondary	Level 1–4
Biceps curl	Sit on a bench	Two dumbbells	Reverse	N/A	Seated reverse-grip dumbbell curl	Secondary only	Level 1–4
Biceps curl	Sit on a bench	Two dumbbells	Palms facing each other	N/A	Seated hammer curl	Primary or secondary	Level 1–4
Biceps curl	Sit on a bench	Two dumbbells	Palms facing each other	Twist wrists as you curl	Seated twisting dumbbell curl	Primary or secondary	Level 1–4
Biceps curl	Sit on a bench	Resistance bands	Normal	N/A	Seated stretch cord curl	Primary or secondary	Level 1–4
Biceps curl	Sit on a bench	Resistance bands	Reverse	N/A	Seated reverse-grip stretch cord curl	Secondary only	Level 1–4
Biceps curl	Sit on a bench	Resistance bands	Palms facing each other	N/A	Seated stretch cord hammer curl	Primary or secondary	Level 1–4
Biceps curl	Sit on a bench	Resistance bands	Palms facing each other	Twist wrists as you curl	Seated twisting stretch cord curl	Primary or secondary	Level 1–4

The Lucky Thirteen Move	Posture Spin-Off	Tool Spin-Off	Grip Spin-Off	Here's a Twist	Here's What You've Just Created	Here's What Type of Exercise It Is	Who Should Do It?
Biceps curl	Lie on an incline bench	Two dumbbells	Normal	N/A	Incline dumbbell curl	Primary or secondary	Level 1–4
Biceps curl	Lie on an incline bench	Two dumbbells	Reverse	N/A	Incline reverse-grip dumbbell curl	Secondary only	Level 1–4
Biceps curl	Lie on an incline bench	Two dumbbells	Palms facing each other	N/A	Incline hammer curl	Primary or secondary	Level 1–4
Biceps curl	Lie on an incline bench	Two dumbbells	Palms facing each other	Twist wrists as you curl	Incline twisting curl	Primary or secondary	Level 1–4
Biceps curl	Lie on an incline bench	Resistance bands	Normal	N/A	Incline stretch cord curl	Primary or secondary	Level 1–4
Biceps curl	Lie on an incline bench	Resistance bands	Reverse	N/A	Incline reverse stretch cord hammer curl	Secondary only	Level 1–4
Biceps curl	Lie on an incline bench	Resistance bands	Palms facing each other	N/A	Incline stretch cord hammer curl	Primary or secondary	Level 1–4

SITTING ON A BALL

The Lucky Thirteen Move	Posture Spin-Off	Tool Spin-Off	Grip Spin-Off	Here's a Twist	Here's What You've Just Created	Here's What Type of Exercise It Is	Who Should Do It?
Biceps curl	Sit on a ball	Two dumbbells	Normal	N/A	Stability ball curl	Primary or secondary	Level 2–4
Biceps curl	Sit on a ball	Two dumbbells	Reverse	N/A	Stability ball reverse curl	Secondary only	Level 2–4
Biceps curl	Sit on a ball	Two dumbbells	Palms facing each other	N/A	Stability ball hammer curl	Primary or secondary	Level 2–4
Biceps curl	Sit on a ball	Two dumbbells	Palms facing each other	Twist wrists as you curl	Stability ball twisting curl	Primary or secondary	Level 2–4
Biceps curl	Sit on a ball	Resistance bands	Normal	N/A	Stability ball stretch cord curl	Primary or secondary	Level 2–4
Biceps curl	Sit on a ball	Resistance bands	Reverse	N/A	Stability ball stretch cord reverse curl	Secondary only	Level 2–4
Biceps curl	Sit on a ball	Resistance bands	Palms facing each other	N/A	Stability ball stretch cord hammer curl	Primary or secondary	Level 2–4
Biceps curl	Sit on a ball	Resistance bands	Palms facing each other	Twist wrists as you curl	Stability ball stretch cord twisting curl	Primary or secondary	Level 2–4

The Lucky Thirteen Move	Posture Spin-Off	Tool Spin-Off	Grip Spin-Off	Here's a Twist	Here's What You've Just Created	Here's What Type of Exercise It Is	Who Should Do It?
Biceps curl	Sit on a preacher bench	Barbell	Normal	N/A	Barbell preacher curl	Primary or secondary	Level 1–4
Biceps curl	Sit on a preacher bench	Barbell	Reverse	N/A	Reverse-grip barbell preacher curl	Secondary only	Level 1–4
Biceps curl	Sit on a preacher bench	Two dumbells	Normal	N/A	Dumbbell preacher curl	Primary or secondary	Level 1–4
Biceps curl	Sit on a preacher bench	Two dumbells	Reverse	N/A	Dumbbell reverse-grip preacher curl	Secondary only	Level 1–4
Biceps curl	Sit on a preacher bench	Two dumbells	Palms facing each other	N/A	Dumbbell preacher hammer curl	Primary or secondary	Level 1–4
Biceps curl	Sit on a preacher bench	One dumbell	Normal	N/A	One-arm dumbbell preacher curl	Primary or secondary	Level 1–4
Biceps curl	Sit on a preacher bench	One dumbell	Reverse	N/A	One-arm reverse-grip dumbbell preacher curl	Secondary only	Level 1–4
Biceps curl	Sit on a preacher bench	One dumbell	Palm facing in	hammer N/A	One-arm preacher curl	Primary or secondary	Level 1–4
Biceps curl	Sit on a preacher bench	One-hand low-cable pulley	Normal	N/A	One-hand preacher cable curl	Primary or secondary	Level 1–4
Biceps curl	Sit on a preacher bench	One-hand low-cable pulley	Reverse	N/A	One-hand preacher reverse cable curl	Secondary only	Level 1–4
Biceps curl	Sit on a preacher bench	One-hand low-cable pulley	Palm facing in	Attach a rope to the pulley	One-hand preacher rope curl	Secondary only	Level 1–4

The Lucky Thirteen Move	Posture Spin-Off	Tool Spin-Off	Grip Spin-Off	Here's a Twist	Here's What You've Just Created	Here's What Type of Exercise It Is	Who Should Do It?
Biceps curl	Sit on a preacher bench	Two-hand low-cable pulley	Normal	N/A	Two-hand preacher cable curl	Primary or secondary	Level 1–4
Biceps curl	Sit on a preacher bench	Two-hand low-cable pulley	Reverse	N/A	Two-hand preacher reverse cable curl	Secondary only	Level 1–4
Biceps curl	Sit on a preacher bench	Two-hand low-cable pulley	Palms facing each other	Attach a rope to the pulley	Two-hand preacher rope curl	Primary or secondary	Level 1–4
Biceps curl	Sit on a preacher bench	Resistance bands	Normal	N/A	Stretch cord preacher curl	Primary or secondary	Level 1–4
Biceps curl	Sit on a preacher bench	Resistance bands	Reverse	N/A	Stretch cord reverse-grip preacher curl	Secondary only	Level 1–4
Biceps curl	Sit on a preacher bench	Resistance bands	Palms facing each other	N/A	Stretch cord preacher hammer curl	Primary or secondary	Level 1–4
Biceps curl	Sit on a preacher bench	E-Z curl bar	Normal	N/A	E-Z bar preacher curl	Primary or secondary	Level 1–4
Biceps curl	Sit on a preacher bench	E-Z curl bar	Wide	N/A	E-Z bar wide-grip preacher curl	Primary or secondary	Level 3–4
Biceps curl	Sit on a preacher bench	E-Z curl bar	Close	N/A	E-Z bar close-grip preacher curl	Primary or secondary	Level 3–4
Biceps curl	Sit on a preacher bench	E-Z curl bar	Reverse	N/A	E-Z bar reverse-grip preacher curl	Secondary only	Level 1–4

12. SPIN-OFF OF THE CRUNCH

SPIN-OFF 1: CHANGE YOUR POSTURE

The Lucky Thirteen Posture: Lying on Floor
(Legs Bent at Ninety-Degree Angles, Feet Flat on Floor)

Posture Spin-Off 1: Lying on Floor (Legs Bent, Feet Up)

For this spin-off, your legs will still be bent at ninety-degree angles, only you'll raise your legs up until your thighs are perpendicular to the floor. If you're looking for more of a challenge, you can keep your legs bent at ninety degrees, but raise your feet just a few inches off the floor.

Whichever spin-off you decide to use, you'll keep your legs in this position throughout the entire exercise (unless I throw you a twist to try).

Posture Spin-off 2: Lying on a Slant Board

Sit on an incline sit-up board and hook your legs into the rollers for support. Lie down so that your head, neck, and back are supported by the bench and place your hands by your ears. Now, slowly curl your head and shoulders forward and up off the bench, then lower yourself back down.

Posture Spin-Off 3: Lying on a Stability Ball

Sit on a stability ball with your legs bent, feet flat on the floor. Keeping your feet in place, slowly lean back and roll yourself down the ball until your shoulders and back are the only things touching the ball. Slowly curl yourself up off the ball, keeping the ball steady as you go, then lower yourself back down. Give yourself plenty of room to either side the first couple of times you do these just in case you fall off!

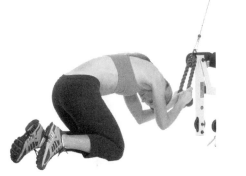
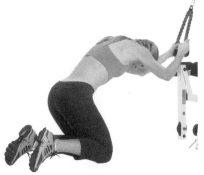

Posture Spin-Off 4: Seated

Place a bench right in front of a high-cable pulley, sit down facing the exercise station, and grab the pulley above you. Bring your hands toward your forehead holding the pulley handle with palms toward the back, then crunch down only as far as you would lying flat on the floor. Don't have a bench? You can always kneel in front of the high-cable pulley instead.

SPIN-OFF 2: CHANGE YOUR TOOLS

The Lucky Thirteen Tool: Just Your Body Weight

Tool Spin-Off 1: Weight Plate
For this spin-off, you'll be holding the weight plate with both hands.

Tool Spin-Off 2: Medicine Ball
For this spin-off, you'll be holding the ball with both hands.

Tool Spin-Off 3. One Dumbbell
For this spin-off, you'll be holding a single dumbbell by its ends with both hands.

Tool Spin-Off 4: Two-Hand Low-Cable Pulley
For this spin-off, attach a double rope to the pulley and grab one end in each hand. You'll need to lie down so that the rope is behind you; that way, you'll feel tension from the cable as you curl up holding the rope ends.

Tool Spin-Off 5: Two-Hand High-Cable Pulley
You can use this spin-off from a seated or standing posture. For this spin-off, attach a rope to the high-cable pulley and grab one end in each hand. You should feel the tension com-

ing from above you as you crunch your torso down toward the floor. You can face the cable or face away from it. Try to bend by contracting the abdominals and not just from the waist using momentum. Try to feel the contraction.

Tool Spin-Off 6: Resistance Bands

For this spin-off, tie or fasten the resistance bands to a low sturdy object and grab one end in each hand. You'll need to lie down so that the bands are behind you coming over your shoulders; that way, you'll feel tension from them as you curl up.

SPIN-OFF 3: CHANGE YOUR GRIP

The Lucky Thirteen Grip: Hands by Ears

Grip Spin-Off 1:Hands by Chest, Elbows Bent

This spin-off is used often when you use a weight plate, dumbbell, medicine ball, etc. If you're asked to use this grip spin-off and you're also asked to hold something, then place that object across the upper part of your chest and hold it with both hands, keeping your elbows out to your sides. If there is no tool spin-off, then just place your hands comfortably on your chest throughout the exercise.

Grip Spin-Off 2: Arms Extended, Upper Arms Alongside Your Ears

This spin-off has you reaching behind you so that your arms are in line with your head. As you curl upward, keep your arms in place throughout the exercise (with your upper arms nearly touching your ears) until I throw you a twist.

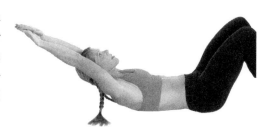

The Twists to Expect

Extend your arms forward

If your hands are over your head, then sweep your arms up and forward so that your hands end up over your knees as you crunch up. If your hands are on your chest or holding something by your chest, extend your arms (and the object) so that your hands point over your knees as you crunch up.

Throw

You'll only be using this twist when your tool spin-off is a medicine ball and you have a partner to catch the ball for you, or when you're trying to get kicked out of your gym. Depending on where the exercise has your arms placed, you'll be throwing the ball either forward, to the left, or to the right. Stay in your "crunched-up" position until your partner tosses the ball back to you, then crunch back down, bringing your hands back to the starting position of the exercise.

Twist from side to side

In *all* of the positions, you can twist to the left and right instead of just curling straight up. This twist brings more of your obliques (the "love handle" muscles along the sides of your torso) into the movement.

READY TO TAKE CHARGE OF YOUR WORKOUTS?

Thought you knew only a handful of exercises to work your abdominals? Look at what you can do now!

The Lucky Thirteen Move	Posture Spin-Off	Tool Spin-Off	Grip Spin-Off	Here's a Twist	Here's What You've Just Created	Here's What Type of Exercise It Is	Who Should Do It?
Crunch	Lie flat, feet on floor or feet up	None	Hands by ears	N/A	Crunch 1	Primary or secondary	Level 1–4
Crunch	Lie flat, feet on floor or feet up	None	Hands by chest	N/A	Crunch 2	Primary or secondary	Level 1–4
Crunch	Lie flat, feet on floor or feet up	None	Hands by chest	Extend your arms forward	Reaching crunch	Primary or secondary	Level 1–4
Crunch	Lie flat, feet on floor or feet up	None	Arms above head	N/A	Long-arm crunch	Primary or secondary	Level 2–4
Crunch	Lie flat, feet on floor or feet up	None	Arms above head	Extend your arms forward	Long-arm reaching crunch	Primary or secondary	Level 2–4
Crunch	Lie flat, feet on floor or feet up	One dumbbell	Hands by chest	N/A	Dumbbell crunch	Primary or secondary	Level 2–4
Crunch	Lie flat, feet on floor or feet up	One dumbbell	Hands by chest	Extend your arms forward	Reaching dumbbell crunch	Primary or secondary	Level 2–4
Crunch	Lie flat, feet on floor or feet up	One dumbbell	Arms above head	N/A	Long-arm dumbbell crunch	Primary or secondary	Level 3–4
Crunch	Lie flat, feet on floor or feet up	Weight plate	Hands by chest	N/A	Weighted crunch	Primary or secondary	Level 2–4
Crunch	Lie flat, feet on floor or feet up	Weight plate	Arms above head	N/A	Long-arm weighted crunch	Primary or secondary	Level 3–4
Crunch	Lie flat, feet on floor or feet up	Two-hand low-cable pulley	Hands by ears	N/A	Two-handed cable crunch 1	Primary or secondary	Level 2–4
Crunch	Lie flat, feet on floor or feet up	Two-hand low-cable pulley	Hands by chest	N/A	Two-handed cable crunch 2	Primary or secondary	Level 2–4

The Lucky Thirteen Move	Posture Spin-Off	Tool Spin-Off	Grip Spin-Off	Here's a Twist	Here's What You've Just Created	Here's What Type of Exercise It Is	Who Should Do It?
Crunch	Lie flat, feet on floor or feet up	Medicine ball	Hands by chest	N/A	Medicine ball crunch	Primary or secondary	Level 2–4
Crunch	Lie flat, feet on floor or feet up	Medicine ball	Hands by chest	Extend your arms forward	Medicine ball reaching crunch	Primary or secondary	Level 2–4
Crunch	Lie flat, feet on floor or feet up	Medicine ball	Arms above head	N/A	Medicine ball long-arm crunch	Primary or secondary	Level 3–4
Crunch	Lie flat, feet on floor or feet up	Medicine ball	Arms above head	Extend your arms forward	Medicine ball long-arm reaching crunch	Primary or secondary	Level 3–4
Crunch	Lie flat, feet on floor or feet up	Medicine ball	Arms above head	Extend your arms forward/throw	Medicine ball reaching crunch	Primary or secondary	Level 3–4
Crunch	Lie flat, feet on floor or feet up	Resistance bands	Hands by ears	N/A	Stretch cord crunch 1	Primary or secondary	Level 2–4
Crunch	Lie flat, feet on floor or feet up	Resistance bands	Hands by chest	N/A	Stretch cord crunch 2	Primary or secondary	Level 2–4
Crunch	Lie flat, feet on floor or feet up	All of the above variations	All of the above variations	Twist from side to side	Use above name with "twisting"	Primary or secondary	Same as original move

LYING ON A SLANT BOARD

The Lucky Thirteen Move	Posture Spin-Off	Tool Spin-Off	Grip Spin-Off	Here's a Twist	Here's What You've Just Created	Here's What Type of Exercise It Is	Who Should Do It?
Crunch	Lie on a slant board	None	Hands by ears	N/A	Decline crunch 1	Primary or secondary	Level 2–4
Crunch	Lie on a slant board	None	Hands by chest	N/A	Decline crunch 2	Primary or secondary	Level 2–4
Crunch	Lie on a slant board	None	Hands by chest	Extend your arms forward	Decline reaching crunch	Primary or secondary	Level 2–4
Crunch	Lie on a slant board	One dumbbell	Hands by chest	N/A	Decline dumbbell crunch	Primary or secondary	Level 2–4
Crunch	Lie on a slant board	One dumbbell	Hands by chest	Extend your arms forward	Decline reaching dumbbell crunch	Primary or secondary	Level 2–4
Crunch	Lie on a slant board	Weight plate	Hands by chest	N/A	Decline weighted crunch	Primary or secondary	Level 2–4
Crunch	Lie on a slant board	Two-hand low-cable pulley	Hands by ears	N/A	Decline two-handed cable crunch 1	Primary or secondary	Level 2–4
Crunch	Lie on a slant board	Two-hand low-cable pulley	Hands by chest	N/A	Decline two-handed cable crunch 2	Primary or secondary	Level 2–4
Crunch	Lie on a slant board	Medicine ball	Hands by chest	N/A	Decline medicine ball crunch	Primary or secondary	Level 2–4
Crunch	Lie on a slant board	Medicine ball	Hands by chest	Extend your arms forward	Decline medicine ball reaching crunch	Primary or secondary	Level 2–4
Crunch	Lie on a slant board	Resistance bands	Hands by ears	N/A	Decline stretch cord crunch 1	Primary or secondary	Level 2–4
Crunch	Lie on a slant board	Resistance bands	Hands by chest	N/A	Decline stretch cord crunch 2	Primary or secondary	Level 2–4
Crunch	Lie on a slant board	All of the above variations	All of the above variations	Twist from side to side	Use above name with "twisting"	Primary or secondary	Same as original move

LYING ON A STABILITY BALL

The Lucky Thirteen Move	Posture Spin-Off	Tool Spin-Off	Grip Spin-Off	Here's a Twist	Here's What You've Just Created	Here's What Type of Exercise It Is	Who Should Do It?
Crunch	Lie on a ball	None	Hands by ears	N/A	Stability ball crunch 1	Primary or secondary	Level 2–4
Crunch	Lie on a ball	None	Hands by chest	N/A	Stability ball crunch 2	Primary or secondary	Level 2–4
Crunch	Lie on a ball	None	Hands by chest	Extend your arms forward	Stability ball reaching crunch	Primary or secondary	Level 2–4
Crunch	Lie on a ball	None	Arms above head	N/A	Stability ball long-arm crunch	Primary or secondary	Level 2–4
Crunch	Lie on a ball	None	Arms above head	Extend your arms forward	Stability ball long-arm reaching crunch	Primary or secondary	Level 2–4
Crunch	Lie on a ball	One dumbbell	Hands by chest	N/A	Stability ball dumbbell crunch	Primary or secondary	Level 2–4
Crunch	Lie on a ball	One dumbbell	Hands by chest	Extend your arms forward	Stability ball reaching dumbbell crunch	Primary or secondary	Level 2–4
Crunch	Lie on a ball	One dumbbell	Arms above head	N/A	Stability ball long-arm dumbbell crunch	Primary or secondary	Level 3–4
Crunch	Lie on a ball	Weight plate	Hands by chest	N/A	Stability ball weighted crunch	Primary or secondary	Level 2–4
Crunch	Lie on a ball	Weight plate	Arms above head	N/A	Stability ball long-arm weighted crunch	Primary or secondary	Level 3–4

The Lucky Thirteen Move	Posture Spin-Off	Tool Spin-Off	Grip Spin-Off	Here's a Twist	Here's What You've Just Created	Here's What Type of Exercise It Is	Who Should Do It?
Crunch	Lie on a ball	Two-hand low-cable pulley	Hands by ears	N/A	Stability ball two-handed cable crunch 1	Primary or secondary	Level 2–4
Crunch	Lie on a ball	Two-hand low-cable pulley	Hands by chest	N/A	Stability ball two-handed cable crunch 2	Primary or secondary	Level 2–4
Crunch	Lie on a ball	Medicine ball	Hands by chest	N/A	Stability ball medicine ball crunch	Primary or secondary	Level 2–4
Crunch	Lie on a ball	Medicine ball	Hands by chest	Extend your arms forward	Stability ball medicine ball reaching crunch	Primary or secondary	Level 2–4
Crunch	Lie on a ball	Medicine ball	Arms above head	N/A	Stability ball medicine ball long-arm crunch	Primary or secondary	Level 3–4
Crunch	Lie on a ball	Medicine ball	Arms above head	Extend your arms forward	Stability ball medicine ball reaching long-arm crunch	Primary or secondary	Level 3–4
Crunch	Lie on a ball	Medicine None	Arms above head	Extend your arms forward/throw	Stability ball medicine ball reaching crunch	Primary or secondary	Level 3–4
Crunch	Lie on a ball	Resistance bands	Hands by ears	N/A	Stability ball stretch cord crunch 1	Primary or secondary	Level 2–4
Crunch	Lie on a ball	Resistance bands	Hands by chest	N/A	Stability ball stretch cord crunch 2	Primary or secondary	Level 2–4
Crunch	Lie on a ball	All of the above variations	All of the above variations	Twist from side to side	Use above name with "twisting"	Primary or secondary	Same as original move

KNEELING

The Lucky Thirteen Move	Posture Spin-Off	Tool Spin-Off	Grip Spin-Off	Here's a Twist	Here's What You've Just Created	Here's What Type of Exercise It Is	Who Should Do It?
Crunch	Kneeling	Two-hand high-cable pulley	Hands by ears	N/A	Kneeling cable crunch	Primary or secondary	Level 2–4
Crunch	Kneeling	Above variations	Above variations	Twist from side to side	Use above name with "twisting"	Primary or secondary	Same as original move

13. SPIN-OFF OF THE REVERSE CRUNCH

SPIN-OFF 1: CHANGE YOUR POSTURE

The Lucky Thirteen Posture: Lying on Floor
(Legs Bent, Feet on Floor)
Keeping your knees bent at a ninety-degree angle, you can also raise your legs up until your thighs are perpendicular to the floor. This makes it a bit easier as you've modified the start position.

Posture Spin-Off 1: Lying on Floor (Legs Straight)
Lie flat with your legs straight instead of being bent at ninety degrees. Draw your knees up to your chest, then lower your legs back down by extending them away from you; lightly touch your original position, and then repeat.

Posture Spin-Off 2: Lying on a Slant Board
Sit backward on an incline sit-up board so that your head is flat and resting by the rollers where you would normally place your legs. You'll have to grab the leg rests behind your head with your hands for support. Holding yourself flat against the bench, slowly curl your knees up toward your chest, then lower them back down.

Posture Spin-Off 3: Sitting on a Bench
Sit on the edge of a bench so that just your beee-hind rests on the edge, tucking your hands down behind your glutes to grip the edge of the bench. Now, lean back slightly and straighten your legs almost all the way out, keeping your feet just off the floor. Holding this position, slowly draw your knees up toward your chest (just as you would if doing the exercise on the floor), then straighten your legs back out. You can also do this with the legs slightly more extended and raise them as though you were pushing your shins toward the ceiling.

Posture Spin-Off 4: Hanging from a Bar (Legs Straight)

Hang just as you would to do a chin-up, with your hands shoulder-width apart and your legs hanging straight below you. Slowly raise your knees up toward your chest, but avoid rocking back to use momentum to raise your legs. Lower your legs back down until they are once again hanging straight below you.

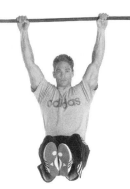

SPIN-OFF 2: CHANGE YOUR TOOLS

The Lucky Thirteen Tool: Just Your Body Weight

Tool Spin-Off 1: Medicine Ball

For this spin-off, tuck the medicine ball between your knees and squeeze your legs together to lock it in place. The extra weight will make it more difficult to draw your knees up to your chest.

SPIN-OFF 3: CHANGE YOUR GRIP

The Lucky Thirteen Grip: Hands on Ears

Grip Spin-Off 1: Arms "Out" from Your Sides, Palms Flat on the Floor

This spin-off gives you more stability by letting you stretch your arms out to the sides for balance.

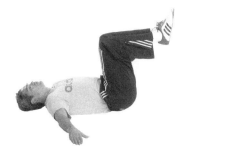 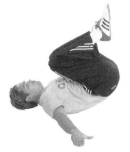

Grip Spin-Off 2: Arms "Down" at Your Sides, Palms Flat on the Floor

This spin-off takes away a bit of your leverage, making the exercise more challenging to your body in order to maintain your balance as you raise your knees (or legs).

Pull in one knee at a time

Instead of drawing in both knees toward your chest, you'll pull in only one knee at a time. Once you've done one repetition, bring your leg back down and draw the opposite knee up.

Raise your legs up

Instead of drawing your knees up toward your chest, keep a slight bend in your knees and raise your legs up until they are perpendicular to the floor. Your body should look like the letter "L" from the side.

Crunch up and hold it

In many of the positions, you can curl your head and shoulders up at the same time as your lower body moves just as you would doing a crunch.

Twist from side to side

In *all* of the positions, you can twist your knees to the left or right instead of just curling them straight up to your chest. Rotating your lower body as you raise your knees or legs brings more of your obliques (the "love handle" muscles along the sides of your waist) into the movement. Keep the abdominals engaged as you add the twist. This is not the time to "let it all hang out."

READY TO TAKE CHARGE OF YOUR WORKOUTS?

Thought you knew only a handful of exercises to work your abdominals? Look at what you can do now!

LYING FLAT ON THE FLOOR,
FEET EITHER ON THE FLOOR OR UP

The Lucky Thirteen Move	Posture Spin-Off	Tool Spin-Off	Grip Spin-Off	Here's a Twist	Here's What You've Just Created	Here's What Type of Exercise It Is	Who Should Do It?
Reverse Crunch	Lie flat, feet on floor or feet up	N/A	Arms out to sides	N/A	Reverse crunch 1	Primary or secondary	Level 1–4
Reverse Crunch	Lie flat, feet on floor or feet up	N/A	Arms out to sides	Pull in one knee at a time	Single-knee reverse crunch 1	Primary or secondary	Level 1–4
Reverse Crunch	Lie flat, feet on floor or feet up	N/A	Arms down along your sides	N/A	Reverse crunch 2	Secondary only	Level 1–4
Reverse Crunch	Lie flat, feet on floor or feet up	N/A	Arms down along your sides	Pull in one knee at a time	Single-knee reverse crunch 2	Primary or secondary	Level 1–4
Reverse Crunch	Lie flat, feet on floor or feet up	Medicine ball	Arms out to sides	N/A	Weighted reverse crunch 1	Primary or secondary	Level 2–4
Reverse Crunch	Lie flat, feet on floor or feet up	Medicine ball	Arms down along your sides	N/A	Weighted reverse crunch 2	Secondary only	Level 2–4
Reverse Crunch	Lie flat, feet on floor or feet up	All of the above variations	Hands on ears	Crunch up and hold it	Use above name with "crunch and..."	Primary or secondary	Level 2–4
Reverse Crunch	Lie flat, feet on floor or feet up	All of the above variations	All of the above variations	Twist from side to side	Use above name with "twisting"	Primary or secondary	Same as original move

LYING FLAT ON THE FLOOR, LEGS STRAIGHT

The Lucky Thirteen Move	Posture Spin-Off	Tool Spin-Off	Grip Spin-Off	Here's a Twist	Here's What You've Just Created	Here's What Type of Exercise It Is	Who Should Do It?
Reverse Crunch	Lie flat, legs straight	N/A	Arms out to sides	N/A	Knee tuck 1	Primary or secondary	Level 1–4
Reverse Crunch	Lie flat, legs straight	N/A	Arms out to sides	Pull in one knee at a time	Single knee tuck 1	Primary or secondary	Level 1–4
Reverse Crunch	Lie flat, legs straight	N/A	Arms out to sides	Raise your legs up	Leg raise 1	Primary or secondary	Level 3–4
Reverse Crunch	Lie flat, legs straight	N/A	Arms down along your sides	N/A	Knee tuck 2	Secondary only	Level 1–4
Reverse Crunch	Lie flat, legs straight	N/A	Arms down along your sides	Pull in one knee at a time	Single Knee tuck 2	Primary or secondary	Level 1–4
Reverse Crunch	Lie flat, legs straight	N/A	Arms down along your sides	Raise your legs up	Leg raise 2	Secondary only	Level 2–4
Reverse Crunch	Lie flat, legs straight	Medicine ball	Arms out to sides	N/A	Weighted knee tuck 1	Primary or secondary	Level 3–4
Reverse Crunch	Lie flat, legs straight	Medicine ball	Arms down along your sides	N/A	Weighted knee tuck 2	Secondary only	Level 2–4
Reverse Crunch	Lie flat, legs straight	All of the above variations	Hands on ears	Crunch up and hold it	Use above name with "crunch and..."	Primary or secondary	Level 2–4
Reverse Crunch	Lie flat, legs straight	All of the above variations	All of the above variations	Twist from side to side	Use above name with "twisting"	Primary or secondary	Same as original move

LYING ON A SLANT BOARD

The Lucky Thirteen Move	Posture Spin-Off	Tool Spin-Off	Grip Spin-Off	Here's a Twist	Here's What You've Just Created	Here's What Type of Exercise It Is	Who Should Do It?
Reverse Crunch	Lie on a slant board	N/A	N/A (hands holding footrests behind you)	N/A	Incline reverse crunch	Primary or secondary	Level 1–4
Reverse Crunch	Lie on a slant board	N/A	N/A	Pull in one knee at a time	Incline single-knee reverse crunch	Primary or secondary	Level 2–4
Reverse Crunch	Lie on a slant board	N/A	N/A	Raise your legs up	Incline leg raise	Primary or secondary	Level 3–4
Reverse Crunch	Lie on a slant board	Medicine ball	N/A	N/A	Incline medicine ball reverse crunch	Primary or secondary	Level 2–4
Reverse Crunch	Lie on a slant board	All of the above variations	N/A	Twist from side to side	Use above name with "twisting"	Primary or secondary	Same as original move

SITTING ON A BENCH

The Lucky Thirteen Move	Posture Spin-Off	Tool Spin-Off	Grip Spin-Off	Here's a Twist	Here's What You've Just Created	Here's What Type of Exercise It Is	Who Should Do It?
Reverse Crunch	Sit on the bench	N/A	Arms down along your sides	N/A	Seated reverse crunch	Secondary only	Level 2–4
Reverse Crunch	Sit on the bench	N/A	Arms down along your sides	Pull in one knee at a time	Seated single-knee reverse crunch	Secondary only	Level 2–4
Reverse Crunch	Sit on the bench	Medicine ball	Arms down along your sides	N/A	Seated medicine ball reverse crunch	Primary or secondary	Level 3–4
Reverse Crunch	Sit on the bench	All of the above variations	All of the above variations	Twist from side to side	Use above name with "twisting"	Primary or secondary	Same as original move

HANGING FROM A BAR

The Lucky Thirteen Move	Posture Spin-Off	Tool Spin-Off	Grip Spin-Off	Here's a Twist	Here's What You've Just Created	Here's What Type of Exercise It Is	Who Should Do It?
Reverse Crunch	Hang from a bar	N/A	N/A (hands holding bar)	N/A	Hanging knee raise	Primary or secondary	Level 1–4
Reverse Crunch	Hang from a bar	N/A	N/A	Pull in one knee at a time	Hanging single-knee raise	Primary or secondary	Level 2–4
Reverse Crunch	Hang from a bar	N/A	N/A	Raise your legs up	Hanging leg raise	Primary or secondary	Level 3–4
Reverse Crunch	Hang from a bar	Medicine ball	N/A	N/A	Hanging medicine ball knee raise	Primary or secondary	Level 2–4
Reverse Crunch	Hang from a bar	All of the above variations	N/A	Twist from side to side	Use above name with "twisting"	Primary or secondary	Same as original move

The Third Wheel: Nutrition

If you close this book and read the cover, you're going to see something missing. You won't find the letters RN, RD, or even "dietary aid" after my name. I'm not a nutritionist. I can't recite what's on the nutrition label of every can in your cabinets, and I couldn't identify a micronutrient under a microscope if you paid me.

But on the cover you *will* find a picture of a guy who used to adhere to a steady diet of Ho-Ho's, Yodels, Ding Dong's, and whatever silly-sounding, chocolate-based pastry I could cram between my once-chubby cheeks. Oh yes: I was fat for a long time. And now, I'm not. Didn't you read the introduction? But I don't attribute my success, or the success of my clients, to any trendy, "sweeping the nation" diet or overhyped pill or fitness product. My solution for shedding pounds was and is much more simple. After all, eating right really isn't all that complicated. It's a choice, and a conscious, daily choice at that. Making the right choice on a regular basis, and sticking with your choice over time, will get you there. Just ask Red Sox fans.

THE FACTS

Function

Choose to eat the right way and you won't just improve every possible aspect of your health, but you'll make the job of reshaping yourself through exercising that much easier. Choose to eat the wrong way and well, look down. Peek-a-boo! Are your feet playing hide-and-seek with you because of what's hanging over your belt? I'm going to make choosing the right way to eat as simple as possible.

The time-starved, almost-always-on-the-go clients I work with are even more at the mercy of convenience eating than you are. I can't monitor what they do 24/7/365 because I am only with them for the hour that we get in the gym. The other twenty-three hours of the day, I have to trust that they'll make the right choices. When they don't make the right choices, their bodies tell me the minute they are back with me.

Inhale the wrong foods and you can easily prevent your system from operating at its most efficient level especially if you're active. Eat less than enough to counterbalance the extra nutritional requirements your body needs to maintain itself and you'll store the same excess fat you're trying to get rid of because your body thinks it's going to starve, and so it holds onto every calorie in anticipation of not getting any more. Even letting yourself get dehydrated by one percent of your body weight in water can impede your body's metabolism, leading to an imbalance of certain metabolic functions responsible for providing energy by delivering oxygen. Water is one of your best friends! Without enough of it, you'll have less energy, and, with all that you are doing, you can't afford that!

Regardless of what your goals are from exercise, following a few basic nutrition rules of thumb (plus a few of my somewhat unorthodox eating tips) will make this third wheel worth a lot more to your body than you ever thought it could be. And the closer you get to your best you, the more influence this wheel can have.

Foundation

If you're trying to lose weight, calories may represent a guilty pleasure or a great evil to your brain. But to your body, calories are just energy units to be used as fuel.

You wouldn't give your car more gas than it really needed, would you? If you did, all that gas would just overflow and make a dangerous mess all around you, right? That's exactly what happens with your body. When you eat more calories than it needs, the result is overflow—to every place your body holds excess calories (a.k.a fat). It doesn't know you don't want to gain weight, it just sees all those extra calories and assumes you want to store them as energy—meaning fat—for later on.

Stand up and jump an inch or two off the ground. Anything move? For every pound of stored body fat you felt jiggle, all you're really looking at is roughly 3,500 calories. Just 3,500 units of fuel that your body "thinks" it needs to hold onto because you haven't given it any reason to think otherwise. But don't worry. Now that you know *why* you're storing calories, it's going to be easier to convince your body to use them up and stop storing them unnecessarily.

Eating a low-fat, high-fiber diet along with doing aerobic exercise to burn calories and resistance training to maintain lean mass and to naturally boost your metabolism, is the most effective way to lose fat without holding you back from building muscle tissue. But attempting to change your dietary habits all at once is usually too overwhelming for most people to handle. I try not to use the word *diet* because it makes people feel like they're walking on a tightrope—one tiny misstep (see *doughnut*) and they assume that all their hopes and dreams will come crashing down. Diets usually involve a drastic change in your eating habits that you'll eventually grow to resent and will almost inevitably quit.

However, knowing what your body really needs can help you ease into making the right changes until they simply become part of your lifestyle. Let's take a look at some common concerns of people I work with—the answers will help ease you into the nutritional habits that will leave your body looking a lot leaner and lighter.

Calories

How many calories you really *need* to eat every day depends on who you are. I've seen clients who can maintain their body weight on 1,400 calories a day. I have other clients with metabolisms like hummingbirds who are so active they could eat suet at every meal and never put on an ounce of fat. It all depends on everything from your metabolism and level of activity to your age, heritage, gender, what you're putting in your mouth, and *when* you're putting it in your mouth.

Need something to start with? The most common method used by dietitians and other health-care professionals is the Harris-Benedict formula. Break out a calculator and run yourself through these figures, using your sex, age, height, and weight:

Men: 66 + (6.3 x weight in pounds) + (12.9 x height in inches) − (6.8 x age in years)

Women: 655 + (4.3 x weight in pounds) + (4.7 x height in inches) − (4.7 x age in years)

$$655 + 641 + 296 - 273 = 1319$$

The number you're left with is your estimated basal metabolic rate expenditure (or BMR), the minimum number of calories your body needs just to keep you going. Getting to work, typing up that report that was due last Tuesday, racing around trying to find a decent place to eat—these are all extra actions that increase your BMR by around twenty percent. For example, a 35-year-old woman who weighs 140 pounds and stands 5 feet 6 inches would have a BMR of approximately 1,402 calories a day. Multiply this by 120 percent and all she "really" needs to eat every day is 1,683 calories a day. If your goal is to trim down, it's just a matter of eating less and/or burning extra calories through exercise to lose weight.

Be honest with me. And be honest with yourself.

The BMR formula works to a certain degree if you like running numbers like an H&R Block rep in April. However, your BMR can change depending on your level of physical activity, certain medical conditions, and so on. It increases when you're sick or pregnant and decreases with age or when you're not eating right, so it's really only a starting point.

I take a simpler approach that requires less guesswork but a lot of honesty on your part. Just write down everything you eat for a week and don't bother counting calories! I don't want you to try to eat healthier than you normally would. I just want you to eat as if you haven't started to think about your diet yet and write down every single thing and when you ate it. Your eating habits don't really change that much from week to week unless you're on vacation, so once you know what you typically take in, you can easily figure out how many calories you really consume.

Your body, whether it's ten pounds heavier or ten pounds lighter than you want it to be, is the direct result of that number. No matter how scary it is, you need to face that number—and usually, you need to change it. Keep honestly looking at your eating habits and they'll honestly tell you how much you need and don't need to eat. My father gave me advice many years ago before I went into business for myself: "Run the numbers first, be honest with them; they may not be pretty, but they never lie." This applies to your caloric intake as much as it does to your business.

Carbohydrates, Proteins, and Fats

No matter how many calories you need each day, it's important to make sure they don't all come from the same place. Carbohydrates, proteins, and fats are all broken down at different speeds in the body to create a continual flow of caloric energy.

Most nutritionists recommend dividing up your daily carbohydrates, protein, and fat using a ratio of 5:3:2 (respectively). This translates into getting fifty percent of your daily calories from carbohydrates, thirty percent from protein, and twenty percent from fat.

GUNNAR'S TIP

Make Your Bad Foods Harder to Eat

You don't always reach for unhealthful food because it tastes better. Sometimes it's like Everest: You eat it because it's there. And in most cases, little prep time or effort is required. You don't need to tell me why this appeals to those with a hectic lifestyle. If you're going to keep high-fat foods around, choose ones that take a little legwork to prepare, like a small pizza or pastry that you have to make yourself. The more inconvenient you can make the bad foods, the less inclined you'll be to eat as much or go back for seconds. And forget dealing with preparation for your post-midnight snack—you won't want to bother! It's all you can do to floss then . . . You do floss, don't you?!

(Those are caloric percentages, not portion sizes!) You can play with these numbers to a certain degree, but it's still important to keep the right balance of all three types of calories. Too much or too little of any of them can lead to a host of problems.

Although I firmly believe it's impossible to achieve all your goals using nutrition alone and eschewing the other three components of a healthy, functional, attractive body—cardio training, resistance training, and the fourth wheel I'll be showing you soon, which is proper rest—I also know that some people are going to try to get it done by diet alone anyway, no matter what I say.

So instead of preaching *not* to do certain diets, I've found what works like a charm is getting my clients to understand the pros and cons of not eating like I've just recommended. The best eating plan can backfire if it's not in sync with your immediate energy needs, your exercise plan, and your lifestyle. What brings you down three belt sizes may be taking you down in other areas as well, from how much muscle and energy you have to a few internal issues you may not be expecting.

Before you run with the latest trendy diet, take a closer look at what happens to your body when you stray too far away from the 50-30-20 plan.

Not enough carbohydrates

Being too carb-conscious can leave you feeling completely energy-deprived, plus avoiding carbohydrates altogether in an effort to lose body fat can severely limit the amount of insulin your body releases into your system. Although *excess* insulin can cause your body to store fat, normal amounts are necessary to start the metabolic functions that encourage muscle growth.

To make matters worse, eating fewer carbohydrates leaves most protein junkies more susceptible to bingeing on junk foods rich in simple sugars (since maintaining low blood glucose levels for long periods of time forces the system to crave sugar to enhance energy). Lack of carbohydrates also depletes muscle glycogen levels in the body. Over time, your body begins to cannibalize muscle tissue, converting it into the glucose it desperately needs for energy.

The guilty diets: Liquid diets, single-food diets (such as the grapefruit or cabbage soup diet), high-protein diets, and even the 40-30-30 plan (the Zone diet) can all be lacking in adequate carbohydrates.

Too many carbohydrates

It's the trap some weight-obsessed people used to fall into. Many low- or no-fat foods are actually highly processed and heavy with carbohydrates (bagels, pretzels, rice, pasta). These refined carbohydrates—which are stripped of many nutrients to extend their shelf life—raise insulin levels and end up stored as fat.

If you love your carbs, opt for low-glycemic-index foods (carbohydrates that burn slowly) like broccoli, beans, snow peas, cucumbers, plums, peppers, pears, and high-fiber, low-sugar cereals. These types of foods can give your body enough of an insulin response to have an anabolic effect on the muscles without causing it to store excess fat.

The guilty diet: Please, it's called the "American diet." Supermarket shelves are lined with products touting the "no-fat" or "low-fat" promise—most of which may not have any fat but are loaded with carbohydrates.

Not enough protein

Your muscles use protein to repair themselves, so not giving them enough only impairs their ability to heal themselves and become stronger. The average person needs to consume approximately one gram of protein for every kilogram (2.2 pounds) of body weight to build and maintain muscle. However, exercise increases your need for protein considerably. If you're looking to build even bigger muscles and are on a serious program, you may require two grams of protein per kilogram of body weight per day (about one gram per pound daily) or more.

The guilty diets: Many fixed-meal-plan diets tend to be *nutritionally imbalanced* and low in protein, not to mention that some are chock-full of chemicals, additives, and loads—I mean loads—of sodium. Plus, to make matters worse, depending on prepackaged food as a quick and simple fix also reduces your odds of having anything fresh get past your lips. A mixture of all these issues can increase your chances of developing a wide variety of health problems caused from excessive sodium and lack of fiber in your diet, including hypertension and heart disease.

Another diet that could leave you protein-starved is a liquid diet, such as Optifast, Slimfast, and the like. Drinking these nutritionally dense shakes for breakfast, lunch, and dinner may help you restrict your caloric intake to around 600 to 1,000 calories a day, but they may also restrict your protein intake—even if they say the shakes offer loads of it. Also, whenever you liquidate protein, glutamine (an amino acid that helps out with vitamin and mineral absorption and muscle function) becomes unstable within just a few hours. By the time the product reaches the store's shelf, most, if not all, of the glutamine has already been broken down beyond repair, making its nutritional value less than what it claims to be. And some liquid diet drinks can also cause minor or major intestinal problems that may not only impair your performance, but may also require you to set up a "second office" in the restroom at work.

Too much protein

Eating extra protein may be good for fat loss and fortifying your muscles, but devouring the protein equivalent of a small farm animal at each meal is not. Your body can absorb only twenty-five to forty grams of protein in one sitting. That means if you're a 200-pound guy that's eating 200 grams of protein a day to build muscle, you should be breaking up all that protein into six to seven smaller meals throughout the day. Why? Any protein left over in your system is considered an excess of calories and stored as fat. Extra protein also over-works your kidneys and liver, which have to eliminate all the extra nitrogen produced from amino acids, the chemical building blocks that are found in protein.

Not quite sure how many grams you had in a meal? Pay attention to your gas gauge—those around you may do the same. If you notice that you're putting forth an abundance of noxious or *ob*noxious fumes, chances are, you've eaten too much protein at one sitting!

The guilty diet: It's easy to see why the Atkins diet is so popular nowadays. Any program that lets you take in loads of protein-rich meats and practically no vegetables seems like many a dieter's "died and gone to heaven" dream. At least, for five-year-old dieters. How-ever, it's not always a safe bet if protein is all you're eating. Most dieters tend to increase their room for protein-rich meat and dairy products by sacrificing fruits, vegetables, or other carbohydrate-dense foods rich in essential vitamins from their diets.

Not enough fat

You may curse it for making your body look like hell, but without it, your body wouldn't last a minute. Fat protects your organs, regulates your body temperature, keeps your skin and hair healthy, and leaves you feeling fuller after a meal, so you won't be hungry and eat more later. It's also essential for protecting and repairing the walls of each and every cell in your body and absorbing vitamins such as A, D, E, and K.

GUNNAR'S TIP

Rotate What You Eat

If you're already getting a minimum of five to ten servings of fruits and vegetables daily, start rotating which ones you eat each day, rather than eating the same healthful food over and over again. Every fruit and vegetable has its own unique mixture of vitamins and minerals. Eat too much of the same foods and you'll always be deficient in whichever nutrients those foods lack. Switch things around every so often and you'll get a more complete nutrient balance of the entire antioxidant family.

The guilty diet: Many single-food diets, such as the cabbage soup or grapefruit diet, are typically fat-deficient. Diets based around one vegetable or fruit can cause a nutritional imbalance in the body. Eating just cabbage, for example, can prevent your body from getting enough B_1, a vitamin essential in helping your body break down lactic acid to prevent muscle dysfunction. Other missing components, such as essential fatty acids and amino acids, add to the nutritional deficit. Lacking either in your diet prevents your muscles from rebuilding as quickly and forces your body to take longer to recover from exercise.

If that doesn't motivate you to add some variety in your meals, think about this. Sticking with the same repetitive eating plan cheats your body of key nutrients it can get only through eating a diverse, well-balanced diet. The long-term effects of this type of malnutrition can lead to a variety of diseases, from cardiovascular disease to cancer. Men in particular should stay clear of the grapefruit diet, since grapefruit has an effect on the P-450 system of the liver, affecting different enzymes that can increase estrogen levels while decreasing the production of testosterone. Not a good look.

Cabbage, on the other hand, is one of the healthiest foods an athlete can eat to prevent a slump, but only once a day. The more intensely an athlete trains, the more antioxidants he or she loses through activity. If the body isn't fed these important vitamins and minerals (magnesium, coenzyme Q10, and vitamin E), it steals them back from its own bloodstream. This in turn impairs the immune system, making you more susceptible to heart disease and cancer over time.

Too much fat

Hmmm . . . I don't really have to tell you why this is not a good thing, do I? I didn't think so.

Water

Virtually every system in your body relies on water to function properly. It does everything from protecting your joints and organs from shock and injury to minimizing the odds of your developing bladder cancer and kidney stones. Water also acts like a cooling system to regulate your body temperature; helps distribute vitamins, minerals, and other nutrients throughout your body; and is crucial in transferring oxygen throughout your body. Staying hydrated can even leave you feeling fuller, lessening your appetite for your next meal. Water also helps keep your skin looking its best.

If you're thirsty, your body is already dehydrated and has begun trying to regulate itself by taking water from your colon, stomach, and kidneys. All this readjusting comes at an exhaustive price. From an energy standpoint, losing just one to two percent of your body weight in water causes a decrease in your performance of between ten and twenty percent. Who can afford that?

Drink as often as you can

Nutritionists recommend drinking at least eight, eight-ounce glasses of water a day, but that doesn't mean you shouldn't drink more than that, especially if you consume alcohol or caffeine, if you sweat a lot due to environment, activity, or a guilty conscience, or even if you expectorate heavily when you talk. You know who you are! Caffeine and alcohol both have a diuretic effect that pulls water out of your system. On average, it takes about two cups of water to make up for the dehydration caused by a single alcoholic drink or cup of Joe. If you're exercising regularly, the minimum amount you should drink is ten to twelve glasses (roughly ninety-six ounces) a day, drinking an additional eight ounces every fifteen minutes as you work out. If this sounds like a lot, try a flavored water like Propel Fitness water or Gatorade. This decreases boredom, increases hydration, tastes great, and you'll forget it's a requirement.

How's the weather?

Exercising, playing a sport, even spending time in an overheated area can cause you to lose up to a pint of sweat an hour (another two glasses of water) without being aware of it. You can get dehydrated and not know it, since thirst can lag behind the body's needs. To prevent this situation, try to drink four to six ounces of water beforehand and continue drinking six ounces of water every ten to fifteen minutes to keep your water level steady. I know the added bathroom stops are a pain, but the trade-off is well worth it. It's all in the planning, people, it's all in the planning!

YOUR OPTIONS

Freedom

Watching what you eat can be as much fun as waiting for the cable company. I'm saying it can be—but it usually isn't. I know that the prospect of living off of bean sprouts and high-fiber cereals (that taste suspiciously like drywall) is something you're not looking forward to. Good news: Eating right does not mean sacrificing the pleasure of eating foods you like.

There are a few ways to secretly change your eating habits without making any major sacrifices in your diet or clueing anyone in to what you're doing.

Boost your bad foods. The next time you're eating something unhealthy, add in something with real nutritional value. Try substituting valueless toppings for something more substantial—like putting spinach and sun-dried tomatoes instead of lettuce on your burger, for example. Or throw some nuts and seeds on top of your nachos. If you're going to eat poorly anyway, this trick at least boosts the nutritional value of your meals by adding vitamins and minerals, and also adds fiber to your diet to fill you up faster.

Eat all day long. Breaking up your daily caloric intake into smaller increments throughout the day (five to six meals) instead of eating the standard three not only helps curb binges, and it also keeps your blood sugar levels even throughout the day. Larger meals raise your blood sugar, which can trigger an increase in the release of insulin within the bloodstream. Eating the same amount of calories you normally would in smaller doses can keep your body from storing this excess as unwanted fat.

Know when to quit. Brussels sprouts may be a nutritionist's dream, but they're going to help you only if you can get them down and keep them down! Much like exercise, you should pay attention to what you like, because forcing yourself to eat foods you despise only sets you up for failure. Instead of feeling the need to overhaul your diet, stock up on fruits and vegetables you know you'll eat (even if that's a limited few for now). Start exploring when you get bored.

Focus

Now that you know how you should be eating, it's time to get serious about doing it. Here are a few pointers on how to make focusing on the basics of good nutrition a little easier:

Trade in your plate. The next time you sit down with a group of people, offer to set the table and "accidentally" give yourself a plate that's slightly smaller than everyone else's. Most people fill their plates completely out of habit, not because they're that hungry. Less space on your plate means fewer calories in your stomach.

Close your eyes. Not all the way, but just enough so you're squinting at your plate and can just make out all the colors on it. If at least twenty-five to thirty percent of your plate looks green (from vegetables), you're eating healthier than most people. On the other hand, if any portion of your food is green, yet you have no vegetables on your plate, you may want to check and see how long it's been sitting in the back of your fridge.

Work backward. Before you dig into your main course, change the order of how you nibble, and start with the least caloric food on your plate (veggies, then starches, then entrée.) By eating in reverse, chances are you'll consume more low-calorie, high-fiber foods, increasing your odds of filling up on healthier fare beforehand. Drinking a full glass of water will also help you cut back. If you don't finish your meal, anything left on your plate will be the most calorie-rich foods you would have normally eaten first. Nice job!

Eat like your ancestors. When you deep-fry, all bets are off when it comes to eating healthy. Suddenly, your system is bombarded with carcinogenic trans-fatty acids and high amounts of calories. An easy rule to remember: The more processed the food, the less nutritional value you'll find in it.

Instead of thumbing through nutrition books to gauge if something's healthy, ask yourself if what you're eating is something your ancestors had access to. Fill up on fruits, vegetables, meats, and grain-derived foods, all packed with vitamins and minerals. This also ensures that you'll have less room for overprocessed foods (such as pasta, breads, and starches) that tend to be higher in sugar.

Add up how many legs your meal once had. When it comes to meat, the fewer legs the animal had when its name was Bossy or Cluckie, the less fat it has when its name is The House Special. That means always go with fish first, then poultry. If you have to choose pork or beef, go for the leaner cuts, such as the loin and round. (That way, you'll have less obvious fat left on your plate when you trim it off. You are trimming it off, aren't you? Good, I knew you were.) Whichever way you work it, you'll be lowering your intake of fats and low-density lipoprotein (LDL) cholesterol and decreasing your risk of heart disease.

Cover yourself with a multivitamin. Add an antioxidant-rich, multiple vitamin that has at least 100 percent of the recommended daily allowance (RDA) of all your major vitamins and

GUNNAR'S TIP

Gunnar's Tip: Eat Something Green Every Other Bite

To limit how much you eat at every meal and make sure the healthful stuff gets into the line-up, have a forkful of some form of water-laden vegetable (such as zucchini, broccoli, lettuce, spinach, cucumbers) after every forkful of the rest of your meal. Eating vegetables in between bites of other food will mix in extra roughage, which will help to: speed up digestion, preventing your body from absorbing as many calories; fortify your body with additional vitamins, minerals and antioxidative phytochemicals; decrease your risk of obesity, certain types of cancer, gastrointestinal problems, and a host of other diseases.

206 minerals. Nearly all of the reputable vitamin companies fit the bill for both men and women, although older women should look for a multivitamin with extra calcium and vitamin D to protect against bone loss or thinning (osteoporosis). This can help fill in potential potholes in your diet, but make sure to take it first thing in the morning on an empty stomach. Having food inside your stomach can prevent the absorption of those vitamins and minerals your body may desperately need.

Gunnar's Tip: They're Just Like You

Think you're the only one that's ever been clueless about proper nutrition? Think again!

Of all the people I've worked out with over the years, who would I say has been the most clueless about nutrition? That's easy.

Me.

There was only one thing worse than growing up as a fat kid and that was having a brother who wasn't one. My younger brother Tor had always been naturally thin and was able to eat as much as he wanted, not to mention that he was also extremely athletic, freakishly smart, and good-looking—a textbook set-up for sibling envy! The guy would devour peanut butter-and-jelly sandwiches and forty-two-ounce steaks like he was in an eating contest, and he never got fat.

I blamed my metabolism and whined constantly about how unfair it was that I had to worry about my weight while he chowed on high-fat take-out. Then one day, I took a break from complaining about my weight and decided to write down everything I ate. I kept track for an entire week. Finally, at the end of those seven days, I did the math—and the answer was right there in front of me.

I was eating about 5,500 calories a day. This was in college, long after I had mastered, in my mind, Weight Watchers and had moved over to nachos. And pizza. And potato chips. And hot dogs. And beer. It was college, after all.

It was hard, at first, to change the way I thought about myself. I wasn't a victim of a poor metabolism. Instead, I'd clearly been bringing my weight problem on myself. But finally discovering that *I* was really behind what was making me miserable was actually enlightening. There's nowhere to hide when you're all alone and those numbers don't lie. My dad was right.

My hope is that you'll use the advice in this chapter. Discover the same thing about yourself, and finally turn the page on a difficult chapter of your life to regain control. As my NBA clients are wont to say: "Take it to the hoop by yourself."

1. "Won't skipping breakfast help me lose more weight?"

I know people who somehow can find the minutes in the morning to put on elaborate makeup or contour their facial hair, but they tell me they don't have time to eat! You are doing yourself a disservice by skipping breakfast or lunch. Odds are, you're still meeting your caloric requirement by taking in the balance at night. And who do you think you're fooling with this "no time" line? So many options are portable, allowing you to grab and eat on your commute. But that's not really the problem: The problem is that you think you'll avoid the calories altogether by skipping a meal. Not a smart decision. What seems like a surefire way to lose weight actually messes up your body internally.

Not eating breakfast, or skipping any meal for that matter, elicits an emergency response from your body. Missing a meal is interpreted as starvation by your body, causing it to store a larger percentage of what you eat next as fat, even if what you've just eaten was entirely fat-free. Dodging breakfast can also trigger a tremendous craving for large quantities of food later on. In other words, eating less in the morning may cause you to eat more than usual during the day to make up for the lost calories.

2. "What's the best thing to eat to start the day?"

To get the most from your morning, you still need to follow the 50-30-20 plan by choosing a meal that's the right combination of complex carbohydrates and protein. Protein takes approximately four hours to digest, whereas carbohydrates take two hours at the most. Eating both within the same meal increases your alertness by burning calories at staggered times for a constant stream of energy, which is crucial when you're trying to get yourself going. Some examples: oatmeal, Ezekiel bread, dried yams and yogurt or egg whites or lox.

Also, choose bagels or toast made from whole grain over the regular processed variety. Whole-grain breads contain more fiber, extra roughage that can make one portion seem just as satisfying as two portions of their processed versions. If you want to make sure your body has time to feel its effects, eat one half of the bagel, then wait at least thirty minutes to eat the other half.

3. "I drink coffee all day long. Does that count toward staying hydrated?"

Coffee elicits a diuretic response from your body, meaning your body loses water as you drink coffee. You may feel more energized, but hitting the java makes you less hydrated throughout the day. All those high-priced lattes also raise cortisol levels (a hormone released when the body is under stress) for over twelve to fourteen hours. That extra cortisol raises your insulin levels and blood sugar levels, encouraging the storage of any excess calories you've got floating around.

Opt for some fresh-squeezed juice cut with water instead. A high-pulp juice will keep your cortisol levels low, the added water helps keep your blood sugar from spiking, plus all the extra fiber can leave you feeling fuller than that cup of coffee would have.

4. "Should I eat right before I go to bed?"

Stop your snacking at least three hours before bedtime. If you eat right before hitting the sheets, your body is likely to store those calories as unwanted fat. However, going to bed hungry can trigger the same starvation/fat storage response that skipping breakfast creates, encouraging your body to store any excess calories it can find as fat. If you wake up hungry during the night, try turning to celery stalks, broccoli, or any type of steamed vegetables as a midnight snack. You never want to feel hungry, since starving yourself only slows down your metabolism as your body clings to the fuel it has left. And the deprivation usually leads to bingeing, which is even harder on your waistline when your metabolism has slowed to a crawl.

The Fourth Wheel: Rest and Recovery

It sounds like the easiest wheel of the four to drive on, but it's actually the one that most frequently gets either too much or too little use. Give your body too much rest and it'll look like it. Give it too little and you increase your odds of not only injuring yourself, but never seeing the body-shaping results you're shooting for. Not sure where you stand? Here's the deal. . . .

THE FACTS (WHAT YOU NEED TO DO)

Function

Whether you hate or love exercise, your body interprets all that time you've spent pulling, pushing, and sweating on gym equipment as one thing and one thing only: *stress.* That's why the time you give your muscles to rest and recover in between each workout can make a huge difference in the kind of results you end up seeing for all of your hard work.

Getting my clients to take a rest in between sets to let their muscles recharge is easy; getting them to take a breather from some of their other activities to let their muscles recharge is another story. Not giving your body enough recovery time to heal itself after exercise can steadily deplete your body's energy in several ways. The first ties into the obvious physical effort you're continuously putting your body through. When you push your body to the point where it can't recover as well from your workouts, that's called *overtraining* in my business. Not giving your muscles enough downtime can leave them in a constant state of exhaustion, which not only prevents them from getting stronger and shaping any further, but also leaves them weaker than usual. Weaker not just when you exercise, but all day long.

Exercising without proper rest also has an effect on what lies below and over your muscles. Continuous intense exercise exhausts the adrenal glands, resulting in blood sugar imbalances that cause energy levels to ebb and flow in unpredictable ways. Keeping your blood sugar out of whack can also cause your body to step into a "survival mode" that tells it to store more fat. Finally, running full steam all the time imposes on the immune system, making you more susceptible to colds, flus, fatigue, moodiness, persistent muscular soreness, sleep problems, loss of appetite, and a lack of "desire" (I'll leave it to your imagination to figure out why that last one really hits home!).

Foundation

Between Sets

Most people rest for too long between each set in their routines. Waiting longer between sets than it takes your contractor to finish will leave you with his physique if you don't watch it. Resting for too long after doing an exercise can cause your muscles to cool down too soon, increasing your risk of accidentally pulling something while making your entire workout less effective. Creatine phosphate, the fuel your muscles use during anaerobic activity, returns within 30 to 180 seconds, depending on the intensity of the exercise. This downtime also gives your body time to drain your muscles of any leftover lactic acid (a chemical by-product of exercise responsible for that fun, burning sensation you feel in your muscles when you lift). After three minutes, your muscles are as recharged as they're ever going to be. Sitting around any longer just leaves them thinking that your workout is already over.

Instead, I want you to rest only for as long as you have to—and that depends on how hard you push yourself. The heavier the weight, the more time your muscles need to

GUNNAR'S TIP

Low Lights At Night

A few hours before bedtime, try turning down the lights in your home. Exposing yourself to bright lights while you are up gives cues to your brain that it is time to wake up, even if what you really need is a good night's sleep.

recover. On average, a set of eight to twelve repetitions requires a waiting time of no more than sixty seconds. (If you've done twelve to sixteen repetitions, then rest thirty to sixty seconds; for six to eight repetitions, rest two to three minutes.)

Between Workouts

Being an overachiever might be working for you in other aspects of your life, but with resistance training, it's the biggest mistake most overzealous exercisers make. Lifting weights causes microscopic breaks or tears inside your muscle fibers, breaks that trick your body into thinking it's about to go to war. These fibers react by rebuilding their legions to be stronger and firmer for the next battle, that is, if you give them an armistice to start recruiting.

After exhausting a muscle with resistance training exercises, it needs at least forty-eight to seventy-two hours of recovery time in order to heal from all that microscopic damage. If you work out that same muscle before that time, you not only increase your risk of injury, but your muscles won't be able to lift as much weight, which will only hold you back from using enough resistance to make your muscles stronger.

For the beginner, performing a full-body workout that hits all the muscle groups three times a week, with a full day of rest in between each workout, makes it easy to get enough rest, which is exactly what the Lucky Thirteen program is designed to do. The typical three-day plan is usually a Monday–Wednesday–Friday or Tuesday–Thursday–Saturday schedule, but that's entirely up to what works best for you.

Every Day of Your Life

A decent night's sleep is just as important for survival as food, water, and sex, yet it's usually the hardest of the four to get—unless you're a computer programmer, a sci-fi geek, or a comic collector or a sad combination of all three. Then sex would actually be the hardest thing to get. (Don't get angry if this applies to you. I am simply passing on information that my computer programming, sci-fi, comic collector clients told me. . . .)

Statistics have shown that seven out of ten adults get six or fewer hours of sleep each night of the week. Too many people think that sleep is expendable, which is why it's always the first wheel that falls off of the car or gets a flat. In fact, research has shown that sixty-four percent of Americans would choose $2,000 over a month of perfect sleep. No, I don't know if that's after taxes.

How to dodge this train wreck varies from person to person. Most healthy adults need an average of seven to nine hours of sleep a night. However, there are those insane individuals who can conquer the day after a mere five hours of shut-eye. Others can't perform at their peak unless they sleep like every day's a day off. Whatever your cycle is, find it, stick with it, and start counting how many times you catch yourself yawning. Being tired in the first place is your body's foolproof way of letting you know it needs more sleep. Other warning signs include a tendency to be unreasonably irritable with people and having diffi- culty concentrating or remembering facts. At least I think that's what the other signs are; I can't remember right now, and I'll get cranky if you push me.

YOUR OPTIONS

Freedom

Even though I may tell you to rest for sixty seconds between exercises, there are times when shortening that amount of time has its advantages. The principle behind circuit training (which is a series of exercises performed one after another with little or no rest in between) says that circuit training burns about twenty-five percent more calories after a workout than doing the same exercises with rest periods in between. Still, that doesn't mean you have to go from sixty to zero to see a change. Changing your rest time to fifty seconds one week, thirty seconds the next week, forty-five seconds the following week, and so on, can shock your body and cause it to burn more calories using the same exercises each week.

When it comes to sleep, there really aren't endless options on how to hit the sack. But, you are free to do something that most people never realize and that's to throw away your alarm clock. Why? Because you already have a biological clock inside of yourself that's a better judge of when you should go to bed and when you should wake up. Experts say that if you have to use an alarm clock to wake up, then you're already sleep-deprived. If that's you, think about going to bed earlier so that you will naturally wake up around the time that you have to. Personally, I'd keep the alarm clock though, unless you think those "experts" are going to help you find a job if you lose yours because you're always over- sleeping!

Focus

It seems ridiculous to tell you to focus on rest, doesn't it? How can you sleep easy if you're too busy concentrating! But, what I want you to do is focus on what could be preventing you from getting enough rest during the day.

Maybe you've had one of your rare weeks where you've managed to spend some qual- ity time with your bedding. You've gotten so much shut-eye that sheep count you when they sleep, yet you still feel like someone borrowed your body to run a marathon without your permission. Before you blame your bed, there may be a few other things giving you that sense of lost power and energy.

Sometimes that unexplained sluggishness taking you out can't be pinned on any red-eye flights, all-nighters, or living in the same house with twin newborns. Here's how to organize your life to keep those energy-eaters at bay:

1. Avoid caffeinated substances (coffee, chocolate, soft drinks, teas, diet drugs, and certain pain relievers) for at least six hours before bedtime.
2. Stay away from alcohol and nicotine for at least two hours before bedtime. A few belts may make you sleepy, but alcohol prevents REM sleep, making what shut-eye you do end up getting less effective.
3. Exercise for at least twenty to thirty minutes a day to promote sleep, but avoid the intense kind for at least four to six hours before bedtime. Elevating your heart rate may keep you too alert to pass out when you need to.
4. Sleep only when sleepy. If you can't fall asleep within twenty minutes, get up and do something dull until you feel sleepy but avoid turning the tube back on. Exposing yourself to bright light will only tell your brain to stay awake.

FREQUENTLY ASKED QUESTIONS

1. "Can't I just drink more coffee to make up for sleep?"

No. Needing to soak your spinal cord in coffee every morning to jump-start your brain is a sign of fatigue that you probably ignore. Sure, caffeine may help mask that sleepiness for a while by stimulating your nervous system, but your body is still energy-broke. Eventually, your body has no choice but to demand that downtime whenever it can. Once that triple espresso wears off, your body not only goes right back to the lethargic state it was in before

---

GUNNAR'S TIP

The More You Lose, the Better You'll Snooze

Every extra pound you're carrying around is more than just an eyesore, it's another sixteen ounces of effort your body was never designed to support efficiently. However, all that adiposity taxes your body in other ways besides having to lug it around. Fat tissue still requires a constant source of blood in order to stay functional. With only so much blood to go around, this demand can thin out the amount of oxygen distributed to the rest of your body, taxing your cardiovascular system by forcing your heart to work even harder. Give your heart a rest, and you can rest.

the boost, but can plunge even further as a result from working all morning without getting the rest it deserves. It's a sleep-deprivation cycle that's going to catch up with you eventually, so just give in and get some sleep.

2. "If I want to exercise more than three days a week, how do I still give my muscles a full forty-eight- to seventy-two-hour break in between?"

Once you're ready for more serious resistance training, there are dozens of other combinations that let you work out more often than three days a week, yet still avoid working the same muscles in consecutive workouts. For example, you could focus on your pulling muscles (your back and biceps) on day one, your pushing muscles (your chest, shoulders, and triceps) on day two, and your legs and core on day three. By the time you hit day four, your pulling muscles will have had over forty-eight hours to rebuild and be ready for another workout or you could take the day off! Or you could focus on a single body part one day a week—chest on Monday, back on Tuesday, shoulders on Wednesday, biceps and triceps on

GUNNAR'S TIP

Your Morning Is Your Friend!

So, you're not a morning person. Think you're the only one who can't get her rest right? Think again!

One of my favorite clients is an actress who always came for her daily session at noon—that is, until the day she landed the role in an action movie. With her days completely booked for months, she knew the only time she could even think of training with me was at 5 A.M., right before her set call. I'm a firm believer in the studies that show that anyone can alter their sleep rhythms within ten to twenty-one days if they just suck it up and stick with it. She was convinced that she'd never have the energy to pull it off because she was definitely not a morning person, but I knew I was about to see the best results I'd ever gotten from her. She stuck to it and did an incredible job. When you get it done in the morning, it can really set the tone for your whole day.

You may feel wrecked at first, but exercising first thing in your day in my experience, is the most reliable way to prevent the rest of your life from running interference. The later in the day you schedule your exercise, the more likely it is that something will pop up that derails your best-laid plans. This doesn't mean everyone should go to the gym at 5 A.M. It does mean that you should consider scheduling in exercise when *your* day starts.

I think it took my client two weeks to finally adjust, and to this day, she still works out at 7 A.M. as if she's due on the set. I don't know if I'd officially label her a "morning person," but I do see her achieving every personal fitness goal she has ever set for herself.

Thursday, and legs on Friday. Add in abdominal work on Monday and Thursday, and don't
always leave it until the end of your workout.

And don't worry. The last part of this book will show you how to rearrange your workouts around your muscles and their respective recovery time when you're ready to step it up a notch.

3. "I think I may be pushing myself too hard. Is there a fast way to tell?"

Some people can exercise seven days a week and never overtrain; others may burn out like a birthday candle in a wind tunnel from exercising just a few days a week. If you're experiencing cold sores, mild sore throats, or muscle and joint aches regularly, you could be exercising too many days a week.

One quick way to spot overtraining when it hits is by keeping track of your pulse rate every morning. Once you know your average morning pulse, just look for any changes each day. If your morning pulse ever rises more than five beats higher than normal, you may be getting sick or possibly overtraining. Either way, it means your body needs a rest day to recuperate.

4. "What time should I go to bed at night?"

The good news is that it really doesn't matter, so long as you're getting enough sleep and you maintain a regular sleep schedule. Try to go to bed at the same time every night, then wake up at the same time every morning. This sets and stabilizes your internal clock. If you can regulate your sleep patterns, the time you spend sleeping will synchronize itself with the sleepy phase of your biological sleep clock. What will that do?

Well, research has shown that people who maintain a regular sleep schedule are significantly more alert than those who sleep the same amount of time, but change when they go to bed throughout the week. They're also less likely to experience mood shifts on top of that. So unless Grumpy and Sleepy are your favorite dwarfs, treat your sleep like it's an important meeting that you can't afford to miss.

PART III

STICK ING WITH IT

The Basic Lucky Thirteen Plan

It's finally time to drive on all four wheels like. Understanding the basic science behind shaping up isn't that complicated. Now you can put yourself through the same regimen that I would put you through, tracking your own progress and pushing yourself to reach your goals. That's right. You can put on muscle, lose fat, and become your own personal trainer—right now! Sound too good to be true? It's not. It just takes some work and conviction. I know you can handle that.

THE PROGRAM

It's important to work all of your major muscle groups for a complete, balanced look. Your body's too important a piece of equipment to leave a few weak links that could injure you later. Using the Lucky Thirteen will ensure you'll have a strong, well-proportioned body—one that functions well, looks good, and is less prone to injuries down the road.

Eventually, you'll be doing two, three, or even four exercises for each muscle group per workout. But before you can do that, I need to get you completely comfortable with each of these thirteen basic exercises. That's why you'll be starting by doing only *one* set each of the Lucky Thirteen, in the following order, three times a week.

Monday, Wednesday, and Friday

For Your Legs and Butt

Squats (one set of eight to twelve repetitions)

Lunges (one set of eight to twelve repetitions)

For Your Chest

Chest presses (one set of eight to twelve repetitions)

Chest flies (one set of eight to twelve repetitions)

For Your Back

Pulldowns (one set of eight to twelve repetitions)

Rows (one set of eight to twelve repetitions)

For Your Shoulders

Shoulder presses (one set of eight to twelve repetitions)

Raises (one set of eight to twelve repetitions)

For Your Triceps

Pressdowns (one set of eight to twelve repetitions)

Extensions (one set of eight to twelve repetitions)

For Your Biceps

Curls (one set of eight to twelve repetitions)

For Your Abs

Crunches (one set of eight to twelve repetitions)

Reverse crunches (one set of eight to twelve repetitions)

Use Your Resistance Wheel Wisely

First, warm up your muscles with five minutes or more of a low-intensity cardio-vascular exercise. Now you're ready to use some weights. **You are going to love how you feel!**

For a full-body, muscle-building workout, perform each exercise in the order shown for one set, using a weight that causes your muscles to tire between eight and twelve repetitions. In between each set of exercises, give yourself 60 to 120 seconds of rest before moving on to the next exercise. If you need more in the beginning, take it. But try to stay under three minutes as you progress, keep it short and sweet, and the benefits will be yours! As you get stronger, you will need to increase the amount of weight you're lifting to keep the muscles challenged. Once you can do more than twelve repetitions, increase the weight by two and a half to five pounds in that particular exercise until you are able to do it for only eight to twelve repetitions again.

Use Your Aerobic Wheel Wisely

Your aerobic plan goes hand-in-hand with the Lucky Thirteen plan. When you decide to do your cardio work is entirely up to you, so long as you do at least twenty minutes of some form of aerobic exercise three times a week. If you have the time to do it on your resistance-training days, then save it for after you've done your weights—since it's safer to tire out after using weights. If you're on a weight loss program, you can also add more aerobic exercise between your resistance-training days. You'll be jump-starting your metabolism five or six days a week, instead of just three. That translates to more calories burned during the course of the week.

Again, to maximize your efforts, you need to exercise hard enough to keep your heart rate within your target heart rate zone for at least twenty minutes or more. Warm up for five minutes at a low level, then raise the intensity for one minute and check your pulse. Count the beats for ten seconds and multiply that number by six. If you are not within your target heart rate zone, adjust the intensity and check again. Once you are in your zone, keep it there. If you can't last twenty minutes when you begin the program, just go for as long as you can. Finish your routine with a five-minute or more cool down.

Use Your Nutrition Wheel Wisely

Before you work out

If you have no energy mid-workout, you won't exercise for as long or as intensely as you should. Working out on a full stomach will only slow you down, but having a light snack beforehand can keep you energized. Stay away from rich foods, since fat takes its own sweet time to digest—a drawn-out process that can starve muscles of blood as you work out. Carbohydrates absorb much faster into the bloodstream, provided you eat them in small doses. The best pre-workout foods for immediate energy are a combination of fast-burning simple and complex carbohydrates or a mixture of protein and carbohydrates. For a multicarb snack, try mixing grains with some fruit: a slice of whole-wheat bread with an apple or a small bowl of oatmeal with raisins are two good options. For a protein/carb snack, go with a tuna sandwich, a chicken salad (you know about the mayo!), or a glass of milk with a piece

FOUR WAYS TO GET MORE FROM
THE LUCKY THIRTEEN MOVES!

1. *Step "right" up to the plate.* Bite the bullet and buy yourself a pair of cross-training shoes. They can improve your posture, which in turn helps your muscles work more efficiently with less risk of injury to your ankles, feet, knees, and even your lower back. Some of the basic exercises from the Lucky Thirteen, such as squats and lunges, require extra ankle support to keep feet stable during the movement. Wearing the wrong footwear can cause your feet to slip or force your ankles to bend in directions that can weaken the tendons inside them over time. Running shoes generally lack lateral stability, forcing your ankles to work harder to keep them from twisting to either side. Basketball shoes, on the other hand, offer good support, but may limit your ankles' range of motion and give you inadequate cushioning for your feet, in case you're actually inspired to run after your workout. Besides, who doesn't feel inspired by a new pair of shoes? If you don't have the proper basics when you're starting out, you'll probably end up paying later.

2. *Two up, two down.* What sounds like a drinking game is actually a mantra to keep in mind at the gym. Most people hurry through their workouts and lift weights like they're in a race, but there's a big downside to rushing through resistance training. Lifting weights too fast allows momentum, and other muscles help out, preventing the muscles you're trying to hit from getting a full workout. Exercising too quickly also makes it easier to let gravity lower the weight for you. The lowering, or eccentric, phase of the lift, is just as important in working a muscle as the raising, or concentric, phase. Spending equal time on both phases can give you more results from the very same exercise. Take two seconds to raise the weight and two seconds to lower it, maintaining a pace that keeps you in total control of the weight at all times.

3. *Breathe, breathe, please breathe.* You're lifting weights, not doing a free water dive. Holding your breath as you lift not only raises your blood pressure, it prevents oxygen from reaching your muscles. It also increases your chances of pulling a Valsalva maneuver, a fancy name for putting yourself in a sleeper hold. Less oxygen to your muscles means less air to the brain, a result that can leave you lightheaded, dizzy, and at risk of passing out mid-workout. Not a good look.

    To prevent this, breathe continuously throughout the entire exercise. Exhale as you lift, press, or pull the weight, and inhale as you reverse the motion. Think "Double E": Exhale on the exertion. But, if that proves too difficult, just make sure you're breathing steadily throughout your sets and reps.

4. *Pick up a pen once in a while.* It's hard enough remembering all of the new area codes, so how do you expect to remember what kind of a workout you had the day before. The fastest way to see results is by challenging your muscles with every workout. That means writing down every detail of each workout (weight used, sets and repetitions completed, total time the workout took, how you felt before and after) so you can look back at those details before your next workout. If you have no sense of what you did before, how will you know if you're pushing yourself enough or too much? It may seem like a monotonous chore, having to write everything down, but I guarantee that your sense of accomplishment will more than make up for it.

of fruit for more immediate energy. Whichever snack you decide to eat, remember, keep your portions smaller the closer you are to "lift-off."

After you work out

Before you wash off the sweat, wash your hands and eat—something small, but something. Working out exhausts the body's inventory of glycogen (stored carbohydrates used for energy), making the job of refilling glycogen its top priority. If there's no food in your system to convert into glycogen, your body starts looking elsewhere to replace that energy. Unfortunately for you, the first place it turns to for food is the muscles you just spent your entire workout trying to build. The result is a body that begins to cannibalize itself for energy, using your muscles as some sort of metabolic convenience store.

Eating immediately afterward also helps you refuel for your next workout, since your body converts glycogen—the fuel you've hopefully used up from exercising—at twice its typical speed within the first fifteen to thirty minutes after exercise. If you can't snack immediately afterward, then eat as soon as you can, even if that's within thirty minutes to an hour after exercise. Even though you'll be replacing glycogen at a more normal pace, your body is still in need of excess calories to convert into energy.

Before, during, and after you work out

Drinking plenty of water may have you using the restroom more than is convenient, but it's important if you want to look better faster. Staying properly hydrated is what makes muscles fuller, while all that H_2O filters out post-exercise toxins left inside your muscles that can slow down how fast your muscles can rebuild themselves. But don't rely on your body to tell you when it needs a drink. Once it tells you by turning the "thirsty" light on, you're already running late.

Right before you exercise, drink about sixteen ounces of water. Then sip six to eight ounces every ten or fifteen minutes during your workout, depending on how full you feel or how many bathroom breaks you've had.

Use your Rest-and-Recovery Wheel wisely

Contrary to popular opinion, your muscles don't transform themselves in the weight room. They change while you're sound asleep, dreaming about three-day weekends. Scheduling your workouts every other day (Monday, Wednesday, and Friday, for example) leaves a perfect forty-eight-hour period of rest between each workout—ample time for your muscles to recuperate, rebuild, and recharge.

Now Stick with It

Beginners should stay with this program for at least four to six weeks before introducing any spin-off exercises (found earlier in this book) into the mix. If you're an intermediate or advanced exerciser, stick with the routine for at least two to four weeks. After that, you'll be ready to raise the bar, so to speak, as well.

Ways to Extend Yourself

Have you ever had to answer the question "Do you know how fast you were going?" or "Do I look fat in this?" Then chances are you've mastered the art of stretching. But not the kind of stretching you need to master, if you want to stay limber and avoid injury. It's incredible how many people skip the stretch because they don't believe in the long-term payoff. If staying injury-free isn't enough to get you pulling and tugging, then what about simply feeling better the next day after you work out?

Stretching your muscles after you exercise not only keeps them pliable, but can also make sure they aren't painfully sore a few days later. Whenever you stretch a muscle, your body responds by increasing the amount of blood in that area, which brings with it more oxygen. Your muscles not only use that oxygen to stay active for longer periods of time afterward, but the oxygen also assists in removing excess lactic acid, lessening your chances of next-day muscle soreness (also known as delayed-onset muscle soreness or DOMS).

Think of stretching as cleaning up after a messy meal and preparing for the next sitting. The mess or waste that is left behind is like what is left in your muscles after your workout (lactic acid). Stretching is like the cleaning up and clearing out. You would never wait a few days to clean up the mess (unless you were in college). You'd clean up after you'd cooked, before you started eating or after you finished eating. By the same token, you wouldn't clean up if there were no mess either, would you? Not unless you were an obsessive-compulsive type. So stretch the same way you clean up—afterward! Not before, like so many people commonly believe. Trying to stretch your muscles when they're cold only makes it easier to injure yourself.

After your workout, this seven-move, seven-minute stretching routine is the perfect damage control plan for keeping your body rocking once you've finished your Lucky Thirteen workout.

FOR YOUR LEGS

1. The Straight-Leg Stretch

Stand in front of a sturdy object that offers several heights to rest your foot (a ladder is ideal). Extend one foot out and place your heel high enough on the ladder to feel a stretch. Don't lean forward or bend your knee. This takes the emphasis away from your hamstrings. Hold for ten seconds, breathe, then switch feet to work the opposite leg. You can do it more than once if you feel you need it.

2. The Figure-Four Stretch

Sit on the floor and straighten your right leg out in front of you. Next, bend your left leg, placing the bottom of your left foot against the inner side of your right thigh. Slowly bend forward and reach toward your right ankle as far as you comfortably can. Hold for five seconds, breathe while you are down there, raise back up, then repeat the stretch three to four more times. Reverse positions to work the left leg.

3. The Classic Runner's Stretch

Stand about four steps from a wall. Shift one leg forward about eight inches, bending it at the knee, while keeping the back leg straight. Now, reach out and put your hands on the wall at about chest height, leaning into it as you continue to keep your back leg straight, heel flat on the floor. As you lean forward, you should feel your muscles stretch from your heel to the back of your knee. Hold it for a count of twenty, then relax and shift positions to get your other leg.

FOR YOUR UPPER BODY

4. The Three-Step Doorway Stretch

Stand in a doorway and grab both sides of the door frame at chest level. Slowly step forward until your arms are straight with your chest up, and you feel a gentle stretch throughout your chest and shoulders. Hold for fifteen seconds, breathing all the while, then step back. Next, lower your hands down the doorway to about waist level, move forward and hold for another fifteen seconds. To finish the stretch, reposition your hands at shoulder level, step forward and hold for a final fifteen seconds. Keep your breathing steady.

5. The Three-Part Torso Stretch

Stand straight and raise your arms over your head. Cross your wrists and turn your hands so that your palms touch. Hold for ten seconds, then release. Next, bring your arms out behind you and clasp your hands together. Straighten your arms, drawing back the shoulder blades, then slowly bend forward at the waist as far as you can. Hold for ten seconds, then return to a standing position. Finish the stretch by bringing your arms in front of you and interlacing your fingers. Extend your arms forward, twisting your hands out so your palms end up facing away from you. Hold for ten seconds, then release. You're still breathing, aren't you?

FOR YOUR ABDOMINALS

6. The Plough Combo

Lie on your back with your arms down by your sides. Bend your knees and draw your legs up and over your body until your toes touch the ground behind your head. If they don't reach, make that your goal for the future. You can put your hands on your calves to assist the stretch. Hold for twenty to thirty seconds, then roll back to the starting position. Next, slide your hands down to your abdominals and begin to slowly inhale as deeply as possible. Your belly should rise, not your chest. Finish by taking ten to twelve deep, controlled breaths to stretch the lungs.

7. The Cobra

Lie on your stomach, placing your hands flat on the ground, shoulder-width apart and even with your ears. Press yourself up, keeping your legs and hips flat on the floor, until your arms are straight. Hold for fifteen to thirty seconds, lower yourself back down, and repeat once more. As you become more flexible, try lowering your hands farther down your body (keep them shoulder-width apart) to increase the stretch.

Know When It's *Really* Time for Change

Here's where it gets rough.

You need you to be critical with yourself every once in a while to make sure the sweat you're working up with the G-Force program is working for you. Are the short-term goals of your purpose being met? What needs to be done to make sure they are? Evaluating yourself brings everything you've done full circle. It's a way of honoring the promises you've made to yourself. It's literally and figuratively taking that "look in the mirror." If you remain honest with the following few questions, and stick to your guns and this program, you can work through anything.

DO YOU KNOW YOURSELF INSIDE AND OUT?

You'll never know how far you've come if you can't remember where you started. Change happens slowly; I may be able to spot progress in someone I'm working with, but when you've done it on your own, sometimes it's harder to let yourself see how much ground you've covered toward achieving your goals.

I don't necessarily believe in the scale, but there are ways to monitor yourself as you start the G-Force program with the same detail-oriented eye that I give my clients. The following tests can help you gauge where your progress is heading. Try any you like (or all of them, if you want), then repeat them whenever you need reassurance that you're improving. But wait at least eight workout sessions in between. It takes a minimum of about three weeks to start seeing any noticeable results.

1. The Speedo test

Pull out the Polaroid camera, stand in front of a full-length mirror in nothing but your swim gear, and snap a photo of yourself. I don't want you to flex, stick anything out, or shove anything back in. I just want you to be you. These pictures may not be pretty, but they'll give you an honest look at yourself and how much you've changed down the road. They can also be hilarious at parties in a few years. Usually, it's the suit. . . .

2. The measurement test

Wrap a tape measure around your waist, arms, chest, thighs, and calves and record the numbers. Just be sure to take these measurements in the same spot every time. Your body's covered with its own assortment of markers that make this easy. Look for anything that won't rub off (a mole, a scar, that Winona Forever tattoo that made sense at the time) and wrap the tape measure around it. I don't do this with my clients because I don't want them too wrapped up in these numbers. But if they ask, I will.

3. The old clothes test

Somewhere in your closet, probably hidden in the corner with everything you hope one day will either come back into style and/or magically resize itself around your body, you will find another test. There will be an outfit you used to be able to wear, and I want you to try it on. "Try" may be the operative word but that's okay because we're making changes. Instead of letting that outfit be a brutal reminder of where you once were, let it be a way to judge just how far you've come and just how far you have to go. Remember, make it work for you, not against you!

ARE YOU CHALLENGING YOURSELF ENOUGH?

It's easy to cheat when the only person you have to answer to is yourself.

Hopefully, having someone like me around can help squeeze a great performance out of you. When we are left on our own, it doesn't always take much to let ourselves slide. We all make deals with ourselves, and often wimp out when faced with something difficult. Missing one or two workouts and closing our eyes during a few important meals may seem like misdemeanors in discipline, but neglect enough pieces of the pie and they add up. This can lead to a body with few results and a mind wondering what went wrong. You need to treat yourself like an investment that you expect a return on in the future. Nurture it, watch it, and watch out for it.

If you're doing it right, exercise will eventually come easier to you, but make no mistake, exercise will never be easy. There's something amiss the day exercise feels easy to you, and it's probably a sign that you've missed out on getting as much out of your workout as you could have. This is fine on occasion, but you can't expect to make progress if you're not challenging yourself. You won't fulfill your purpose if you never challenge yourself. Exercise should never be easy. It can be fun, and I believe it should be. But not easy! There's a reason it's called a "*work*out." Stick with that mantra and exercise will always work with you to reach your goals no matter what.

ARE YOU BEING HONEST ENOUGH?

Your perfect physique takes time.

It's not an overnight thing. It's not some plastic surgery "outpatient" procedure you can do during your lunch hour and be done before your coworkers notice you're not at your desk. Unless you're using something illegal or taking other unhealthy and drastic measures to change yourself, your body can only put on about a half-pound of muscle per week until you reach your genetic limit. As for fat loss, you're only likely to lose between one and two and a half pounds of fat as energy per week if you're doing it the right way, and this rate slows as you progress. If you've lost more weight than that, what you've probably lost is nothing more than excess water or even muscle tissue. Not that that is bad; it's just not fat.

Remember, enjoy the journey, every mile of it. You'll get to the destination and be in a better mood when you get there. I've said it before. There is no magic bullet. You won't see a major change overnight. But you will pick up loose change along your way, and take it from me, all that change adds up fast. Every week that you wait around for that magic bullet that promises you'll lose fifty pounds in a month, you've missed out on actually burning away one to two pounds of fat and putting on a half pound of muscle. Think about how many weeks of your life you've wasted waiting around or trying those magic bullets. Then think about how far you could have come in that time. But don't get mad at yourself—get started!

ARE YOU REWARDING YOURSELF ENOUGH?

Don't miss out on your smaller successes while you are focused on your goal. Sometimes, being caught up chasing a new purpose, setting unrealistic goals, or being too self-critical can leave you completely forgetting that you've accomplished what you set out to do. I want you to enjoy the journey, reward yourself on the way to your purpose, and reward yourself when you finally complete your purpose. This reward doesn't have to be a fudge sundae. It can be a subtle smile when you see yourself in the mirror or treating yourself to that movie no one will see with you. It's that simple.

That goes for the goals you may never reach as well. If you were trying to fit back in to that size 2 dress and only got down to a size 6, you should be excited that you got down to a size 6. If your purpose was to bench 300 pounds, but you only got up to 225 no matter what you tried, I need you to relish that. You need to give yourself credit for everything you did do and not just beat yourself up for what you couldn't or didn't do. Despite everything I've ever learned about fitness and exercise over the years, it's remembering to enjoy the remarkable moments that being in shape will eventually grant you that is the most valuable lesson of all. It's the most crucial thing you can do to ensure you'll always meet your goals, no matter what they are or who you are.

It's also something I'm reminded of every day when I look around my office and see pictures of some of the people I've had the pleasure and good fortune to work with over the years—people who owe a piece of their lives to staying dedicated to exercise on a daily basis. But it's one picture in particular that someone once gave me of herself that always knocks that point home. It wasn't the incredible and beautiful shape she was in at the time the photo was taken, but the words she later wrote on it.

It says, "When I looked like this, I wasn't happy. Looking at it now, I am."

Once you reach that first goal, do me a favor, will you? Realize that you *do* have it, then thank the person who deserves all the credit.

You.

Taking the Thirteen to the Next Level

If you answered yes to all the questions I asked in the last chapter, then you're finally ready to do what it takes to push yourself even harder toward that whole new you.

Stop worrying.

You didn't honestly think I would hit you with all of these fitness pearls and then leave you hanging with no string to make a necklace, did you? Aw, c'mon, I thought you knew me by now! I would *never* do that!

As you now know, just changing a few variables in your workout can mix things up enough to feel different to your muscles. Making the right changes when you seem to be going nowhere will ensure that you'll still be looking like a college coed while the rest of your corn-fed friends are busy shopping for plus-size clothing on their way to see the doctor!

GUNNAR'S TIP

Put Your Feet Up on Occasion

When doing flies, shoulder presses, or light chest presses, bend your legs and prop your feet up on the bench instead of placing them flat on the floor. Having them anchored to the ground makes it easier to arch your back, which positions the body at an angle that lets other muscles help lift up the weight. Keeping them up on the bench locks the body into a posture that puts all the effort directly on the chest muscles. This is a great way to mix things up.

PLATEAU

How You Push!

Barbell goes up. Barbell goes down. Barbell goes up. Barbell goes down.

So, you've finally mastered the technique with all thirteen moves, eh? Great. It wasn't that hard, was it?

Now stop.

There are three different ways your muscles can contract when doing resistance training—positive, negative, and static.

They contract positively as you lift the weight (concentric).

They contract negatively as you lower the weight (eccentric).

Finally, they contract statically when you stop moving the weight and just hold it in a contracted state (isometric).

Doing the Lucky Thirteen the way I showed you will work your muscles in all three ways, but there are ways you can further improve your results. To demonstrate each, I'll use the chest press, but all work with almost any exercise.

PARTIALS (builds extra positive strength)

Put yourself in the starting position of a chest press, arms straight, holding the weights above you. Lower the weights to your chest and press them back up. Now, lower the weights again, but this time, bring them only about a quarter of the way down, then press them back up. Continue to repeat this pattern (one full rep, followed by a quarter rep) for eight to twelve *full* repetitions.

GUNNAR'S TIP: Mix up doing the partial move at the bottom or top of the movement. If you usually need help pushing the weights at the very top, stay with the above approach. If the weights tend to get stuck by your chest, try adding partials at the bottom of the movement.

PROOF

STOP-GO'S (builds static strength)

Start with the weights held above you for five seconds, elbows unlocked. Lower the weights halfway down and pause for another five seconds. Continue to lower the weights until they're at the bottom of the movement (just above the chest) and hold for five seconds. Next, press the weights back up and lower them back down normally for one complete rep (the weights should end up back at your chest). Now, reverse the motion, holding the weights for five seconds just above your chest, five seconds at the midpoint, and five at the top. Do another regular rep (down and up) and you're back at the beginning. Repeat the cycle for a total of eight to twelve full reps.

GUNNAR'S TIP: This plateau-proof technique is so taxing you'll need to lower the amount of weight you normally use to about fifty percent. But don't worry. All that pausing keeps your muscles constantly flexed, so you'll look impressive throughout the exercise. I know that's important to you! You can also vary the hold time: five, four, three, two, you can even vary it within the set itself! Do you see the possibilities here?!

NEGATIVES (emphasis on lowering the weight slowly)

Start with the weights above you and two allegiant friends on opposite sides of the bench. Slowly lower the weights down to your chest for a count of six seconds. Once the weights reach your chest, have your spotters lift the weights back up until your arms are straight (elbows unlocked). Don't bother pushing, just let your porters do all the work. Lower the weights again for a count of six, resisting gravity's pitiless pull yet again. Repeat for eight to twelve repetitions.

GUNNAR'S TIP: This technique lets you use heavier weights than you could normally lift, which can help add more size to your muscles. Very few women I work with—or know, for that matter—go in for negatives on any kind of regular basis. I'm not saying anything, I'm just saying . . .

This next section is all about freedom. It's going to be your guide to mixing and matching the right combination of Lucky Thirteen spin-offs into a program that's tailor-made to your fitness goals. Trust me, once you get comfortable with how to arrange these exercises using these guidelines, you'll be well on your way to designing routines like an expert. You'll also want to share your new knowledge and creativity with others. You'll see why I love what I do. Solving problems, creating new programs, and helping people feel great about themselves every day . . . not bad for a *job*!

In each routine, you'll notice the Lucky Thirteen moves follow a certain sequence. That's because there's a pecking order in terms of which muscle groups you need to work. The best exercise plan is designed to work your larger muscle groups (back, chest, legs, and shoulders) before your smaller muscle groups (triceps, biceps, and abs). The reason? A lot of exercises that work large muscle groups also require smaller muscles to help stabilize your body as you do them. Pre-fatigue those tiny muscles first and they'll fail in the clutch when lifting heavier weights to work the larger muscles. So stick with the order shown.

You also need to keep exercises you'll be using for the same body part in the right order as well. Certain exercises (known as primary exercises) may focus on one muscle group, but still require other muscle groups to help you do the move. Other types of exercises (known as secondary exercises) focus on one muscle group using angles that let you focus strictly on that muscle. Doing a secondary exercise before a primary exercise sometimes has its place in an advanced workout, but to make the Lucky Thirteen system as user-friendly as possible, you'll always start with a primary exercise first.

Weren't you wondering what that second to the last column of each spin-off chart meant? You know, this one?

GUNNAR'S TIP

Slow Things Down a Bit

Instead of raising and lowering your weights in the traditional way (two seconds up–two seconds down), try lowering the weight you typically lift by about forty percent and performing the exercise even more slowly (four to five seconds up and four to five seconds down). Doing a set of an exercise in slow motion works your muscles differently, often taxes them as much as or more than a traditional program, and puts less stress on your joints.

The Lucky Thirteen Move	Posture Spin-Off	Tool Spin-Off	Grip Spin-Off	Here's a Twist	Here's What You've Just Created	Here's What Type of Exercise It Is	Who Should Do It?
Raise	Stand	Two dumbbells	Palms facing each other	N/A	Side lateral raise 1	Primary or secondary	Level 1–4

Letting you know which exercises are primary and secondary is my way of making sure you never use a secondary exercise first. In every program, you'll see each Lucky Thirteen move you'll have to do broken down like this:

The Lucky Thirteen Move	The Type of Move You Should Use	How Many Sets?	How Many Reps?
Chest Press	Primary only	1	10–12

See that column that tells you "the type of move you should use"? That's where all those primary and secondary distinctions come into play.

In the beginner routines, you'll be asked to pick a "primary only" version of each of the Lucky Thirteen moves. If an exercise variation you're thinking of trying from the charts says it's either a "primary or secondary" exercise, that means it can be used anywhere in your workout, so feel free to use it. But if an exercise variation you're thinking of trying says "secondary only," that means it should be used only as a secondary exercise. As you start progressing into the intermediate- and advanced-level routines, you'll be asked to pick more than one version of each Lucky Thirteen move within the same workout, like so:

The Lucky Thirteen Move	The Type of Move You Should Use	How Many Sets?	How Many Reps?
Chest Press	Primary only	1	10–12
Chest Press	Primary or secondary	1	10–12

That's where you'll be able to use any of the few "secondary only" moves that you may find in the charts. Otherwise, whenever you're asked to pick a move that's either "primary or secondary," you can use any move you want (so long as it's not an experienced move that's meant for a higher-level exerciser than you are).

THE G-FORCE PLAN FOR EVERY LEVEL

BEGINNER LEVEL

If you have only two days a week, try this:

WORKOUT 1

Aerobic Training

Twice a week, you'll do twenty minutes of aerobic activity (either after your resistance training or on the days in between). Warm up for five minutes at a low intensity, then perform twenty minutes of aerobic activity within your target heart rate zone. Cool down with five more minutes at a low intensity.

Resistance Training

Warm up with a low-intensity activity for five minutes, then perform each Lucky Thirteen move in the order given, resting sixty to ninety seconds between each set.

When to Change

Stick with this program for three to four weeks. Afterward, substitute each of the Lucky Thirteen exercises you've been using for another variation.

MONDAYS AND THURSDAYS

The Lucky Thirteen Move	The Type of Move You Should Use	How Many Sets?	How Many Reps?
Squat	Primary only	1	10–12
Lunge	Primary only	1	10–12
Chest press	Primary only	1	10–12
Chest fly	Primary only	1	10–12
Pulldown	Primary only	1	10–12
Row	Primary only	1	10–12
Shoulder press	Primary only	1	10–12
Raise	Primary only	1	10–12
Pressdown	Primary only	1	10–12
Extension	Primary only	1	10–12
Curl	Primary only	1	10–12
Crunch	Primary only	1	10–15
Reverse crunch	Primary only	1	10–15
		TOTAL SETS: 13	

If you have only three days a week, try this:

WORKOUT 2

Aerobic Training

Three times a week, you'll do twenty minutes of aerobic activity (either after your resistance training or on the days in between). Warm up for five minutes at a low intensity, then perform twenty minutes of aerobic activity within your target heart rate zone. Cool down with five more minutes at a low intensity.

Resistance Training

Warm up with a low intensity activity for five minutes, then perform each Lucky Thirteen move in the order given, resting sixty to ninety seconds between each set.

When to Change

Stick with this program for three to four weeks. Afterward, substitute each of the Lucky Thirteen exercises you've been using for another variation.

The Lucky Thirteen Move	The Type of Move You Should Use	How Many Sets?	How Many Reps?
Squat	Primary only	1	10–12
Lunge	Primary only	1	10–12
Chest press	Primary only	1	10–12
Chest fly	Primary only	1	10–12
Pulldown	Primary only	1	10–12
Row	Primary only	1	10–12
Shoulder press	Primary only	1	10–12
Raise	Primary only	1	10–12
Pressdown	Primary only	1	10–12
Extension	Primary only	1	10–12
Curl	Primary only	1	10–12
Crunch	Primary only	1	10–15
Reverse crunch	Primary only	1	10–15
		TOTAL SETS: 13	

INTERMEDIATE LEVEL

If you have only three days a week, try this:

WORKOUT 1

Aerobic Training

Three times a week, you'll do twenty to thirty minutes of aerobic activity (either after your resistance training or on the days in between). Warm up for five minutes at a low intensity, then perform twenty to thirty minutes of aerobic activity within your target heart rate zone. Cool down with five more minutes at a low intensity.

Resistance Training

You'll alternate between doing the two routines shown (taking Sundays off) and you'll double the number of sets. Each week you'll be repeating one of the workouts. Perform day one, then rest for forty-eight hours. Next, perform day two, then rest again for forty-eight hours. Make sure that before every resistance training session you warm up with a low-intensity activity for five minutes, then perform each Lucky Thirteen move in the order given, resting sixty to ninety seconds between each set.

When to Change

Stick with this program for three to four weeks. Afterward, substitute each of the Lucky Thirteen exercises you've been using for another variation.

4/4, 4/9, 4/14

DAY ONE
(Upper body workout)

The Lucky Thirteen Move	The Type of Move You Should Use	How Many Sets?	How Many Reps?
Chest press	Primary only	2	10–12
Chest fly	Primary only	2	10–12
Pulldown	Primary only	2	10–12
Row	Primary only	2	10–12
Shoulder press	Primary only	2	10–12
Raise	Primary only	2	10–12
Pressdown	Primary only	2	10–12
Extension	Primary only	2	10–12
Curl	Primary only	2	10–12
Crunch	Primary only	2	10–15
Reverse crunch	Primary only	2	10–15

TOTAL SETS 22

4/8, 4/11

DAY TWO
(Lower body workout)

The Lucky Thirteen Move	The Type of Move You Should Use	How Many Sets?	How Many Reps?
Squat	Primary only	3	10–12
Squat	Primary or secondary	3	10–12
Squat	Primary or secondary	3	10–12
Lunge	Primary only	3	10–12
Lunge	Primary or secondary	3	10–12
Lunge	Primary or secondary	3	10–12
Crunch	Primary only	2	10–15
Reverse crunch	Primary only	2	10–15

TOTAL SETS 22

If you have four days a week, try this:

WORKOUT 2

Aerobic Training

Four times a week, you'll do twenty to thirty minutes of aerobic activity (either after your resistance training or on the days in between). Warm up for five minutes at a low intensity, then perform twenty to thirty minutes of aerobic activity within your target heart rate zone. Cool down with five more minutes at a low intensity.

Resistance Training

Warm up with a low-intensity activity for five minutes, then perform each Lucky Thirteen move in the order given, resting sixty to ninety seconds between each set.

When to Change

Stick with this program for three to four weeks. Afterward, substitute each of the Lucky Thirteen exercises you've been using with another variation.

MONDAYS AND THURSDAYS
(Legs, back, biceps, and lower abs)

The Lucky Thirteen Move	The Type of Move You Should Use	How Many Sets?	How Many Reps?
Squat	Primary only	4	10–12
Lunge	Primary only	3	10–12
Pulldown	Primary only	3	10–12
Row	Primary only	3	10–12
Curl	Primary only	2	10–12
Curl	Primary or secondary	2	10–12
Crunch	Primary only	2	10–15
Reverse crunch	Primary only	2	10–15
		TOTAL SETS 21	

TUESDAYS AND FRIDAYS
(Chest, shoulders, triceps, and abs)

The Lucky Thirteen Move	The Type of Move You Should Use	How Many Sets?	How Many Reps?
Chest press	Primary only	3	10–12
Chest fly	Primary only	3	10–12
Shoulder press	Primary only	3	10–12
Raise	Primary only	3	10–12
Pressdown	Primary only	2	10–12
Extension	Primary only	2	10–12
Crunch	Primary only	2	10–15
Reverse crunch	Primary only	2	10–15
		TOTAL SETS 20	

If you have five days a week, try this:

WORKOUT 3

Aerobic Training

Five times a week, you'll do twenty to thirty minutes of aerobic activity (either after your resistance training or on the days in between). Warm up for five minutes at a low intensity, then perform twenty to thirty minutes of aerobic activity within your target heart rate zone. Cool down with five more minutes at a low intensity.

Resistance Training

Warm up with a low-intensity activity for five minutes, then perform each Lucky Thirteen move in the order given, resting sixty to ninety seconds between each set.

When to Change

Stick with this program for three to four weeks. Afterward, substitute each of the Lucky Thirteen exercises you've been using for another variation.

The Lucky Thirteen Move	The Type of Move You Should Use	How Many Sets?	How Many Reps?
Squat	Primary only	3	10–12
Lunge	Primary only	3	10–12

Do both exercises above back-to-back twice more before continuing for a final total of three sets per exercise.

Squat	Primary or secondary	2	10–12
Lunge	Primary or secondary	2	10–12

Do both exercises above back-to-back once more before continuing for a final total of two sets per exercise.

Pressdown	Primary only	3	10–12
Curl	Primary only	3	10–12

Do both exercises above back-to-back twice more before continuing for a final total of three sets per exercise.

Extension	Primary only	2	10–12
Curl	Primary or secondary	2	10–12

Do both exercises above back-to-back once more before continuing for a final total of two sets per exercise.

Crunch	Primary only	2	10–15
Reverse crunch	Primary only	2	10–15

Do both exercises above back-to-back once more for a final total of two sets per exercise.

TOTAL SETS 24

TUESDAYS AND FRIDAYS—PUSH/PULL
(Chest, back, shoulders, and abs)

The Lucky Thirteen Move	The Type of Move You Should Use	How Many Sets?	How Many Reps?
Chest press	Primary only	3	10–12
Row	Primary only	3	10–12

Do both exercises above back-to-back twice more before continuing for a final total of three sets per exercise.

Shoulder press	Primary only	3	10–12
Pulldown	Primary only	3	10–12

Do both exercises above back-to-back twice more before continuing for a final total of three sets per exercise.

Chest fly	Primary only	3	10–12
Raise	Primary only (posture spin-off: bent-over)	3	10–12

Do both exercises above back-to-back twice more before continuing for a final total of three sets per exercise.

Crunch	Primary only	2	10–15
Reverse crunch	Primary only	2	10–15

Do both exercises above back-to-back once more for a final total of two sets per exercise.

TOTAL SETS 22

ADVANCED LEVEL

If you have only four days a week, try this:

WORKOUT 1

Aerobic Training

Four times a week, you'll do thirty to forty-five minutes of aerobic activity (either after your resistance training or on the days in between). Warm up for five minutes at a low intensity, then perform thirty to forty-five minutes of aerobic activity within your target heart rate zone. Cool down with five more minutes at a low intensity.

Resistance Training

Warm up with a low-intensity activity for five minutes, then perform each Lucky Thirteen move in the order given, resting sixty to ninety seconds between each set.

When to Change

Stick with this program for three to four weeks. Afterward, substitute each of the Lucky Thirteen exercises you've been using for another variation.

MONDAYS AND THURSDAYS
(Upper body workout)

The Lucky Thirteen Move	The Type of Move You Should Use	How Many Sets?	How Many Reps?
Chest press	Primary only	2	10–12
Chest fly	Primary only	2	10–12
Pulldown	Primary only	2	10–12
Row	Primary only	2	10–12
Shoulder press	Primary only	2	10–12
Raise	Primary only	2	10–12
Pressdown	Primary only	2	10–12
Extension	Primary only	2	10–12
Curl	Primary only	2	10–12
Crunch	Primary only	2	10–15
Reverse crunch	Primary only	2	10–15
		TOTAL SETS 22	

The Lucky Thirteen Move	The Type of Move You Should Use	How Many Sets?	How Many Reps?
Squat	Primary only	3	10–12
Squat	Primary or secondary	3	10–12
Squat	Primary or secondary	3	10–12
Lunge	Primary only	3	10–12
Lunge	Primary or secondary	3	10–12
Lunge	Primary or secondary	3	10–12
Crunch	Primary only	2	10–15
Reverse crunch	Primary only	2	10–15
		TOTAL SETS 22	

THE

G-FORCE

PLAN

FOR

EVERY

LEVEL

WORKOUT 2

Aerobic Training

Five times a week, you'll do thirty to forty-five minutes of aerobic activity (either after your resistance training or on the days in between). Warm up for five minutes at a low intensity, then perform thirty to forty-five minutes of aerobic activity within your target heart rate zone. Cool down with five more minutes at a low intensity.

Resistance Training

You'll run through all three programs in order, taking Wednesdays and Sundays off. Warm up with a low-intensity activity for five minutes, then perform each Lucky Thirteen move in the order given, resting sixty to ninety seconds between each set.

When to Change

Stick with this program for three to four weeks. Afterward, substitute each of the Lucky Thirteen exercises you've been using with another variation.

DAY #1
(Legs and abs)

The Lucky Thirteen Move	The Type of Move You Should Use	How Many Sets?	How Many Reps?
Squat	Primary only	4	10–12
Squat	Primary or secondary	4	10–12
Lunge	Primary only	4	10–12
Lunge	Primary or secondary	4	10–12
Crunch	Primary only	2	10–15
Reverse crunch	Primary only	2	10–15
		TOTAL SETS 20	

DAY #2
(Chest, shoulders, triceps, and abs)

The Lucky Thirteen Move	The Type of Move You Should Use	How Many Sets?	How Many Reps?
Chest press	Primary only	3	10–12
Chest fly	Primary only	3	10–12
Shoulder press	Primary only	3	10–12
Raise	Primary only	3	10–12
Pressdown	Primary only	3	10–12
Extension	Primary only	3	10–12
Crunch	Primary only	2–3	10–15
Reverse crunch	Primary only	2–3	10–15
		TOTAL SETS 22–24	

DAY #3
(Back, biceps, and abs)

The Lucky Thirteen Move	The Type of Move You Should Use	How Many Sets?	How Many Reps?
Row	Primary only	3	10–12
Row	Primary or secondary	3	10–12
Pulldown	Primary only	3	10–12
Pulldown	Primary or secondary	3	10–12
Curl	Primary only	3	10–12
Curl	Primary or secondary	3	10–12
Crunch	Primary only	2–3	10–15
Reverse crunch	Primary only	2–3	10–15
		TOTAL SETS 22	

WORKOUT 3

Aerobic Training

Six times a week, you'll do thirty to forty-five minutes of aerobic activity (either after your resistance training or on the day in between). Warm up for five minutes at a low intensity, then perform thirty to forty-five minutes of aerobic activity within your target heart rate zone. Cool down with five more minutes at a low intensity.

Resistance Training

Warm up with a low-intensity activity for five minutes, then perform each Lucky Thirteen move in the order given, resting 60 to 120 seconds between each set.

When to Change

Stick with this program for three to four weeks. Afterward, substitute each of the Lucky Thirteen exercises you've been using with another variation.

MONDAYS, WEDNESDAYS, AND FRIDAYS
(Legs, back, biceps, and lower abs)

The Lucky Thirteen Move	The Type of Move You Should Use	How Many Sets?	How Many Reps?
Squat	Primary only	4	10–12
Lunge	Primary only	3	10–12
Pulldown	Primary only	3	10–12
Row	Primary only	3	10–12
Curl	Primary only	2	10–12
Curl	Primary and secondary	2	10–12
Crunch	Primary only	2–3	10–15
Reverse crunch	Primary only	2–3	10–15
		TOTAL SETS 21	

TUESDAYS, THURSDAYS AND SATURDAYS
(Chest, shoulders, triceps, and abs)

The Lucky Thirteen Move	The Type of Move You Should Use	How Many Sets?	How Many Reps?
Chest press	Primary only	3	10–12
Chest fly	Primary only	3	10–12
Shoulder press	Primary only	3	10–12
Raise	Primary only	3	10–12
Pressdown	Primary only	2	10–12
Extension	Primary only	2	10–12
Crunch	Primary only	2–3	10–15
Reverse crunch	Primary only	2–3	10–15
	TOTAL SETS 22		

THE

G-FORCE

PLAN

FOR

EVERY

LEVEL

If you have six days a week, try this:

WORKOUT 4

This workout works each muscle group just once a week. When combined with a diet that provides more calories than what you're burning on a daily basis, this advanced, muscle-building system can help achieve maximum muscle hypertrophy.

Aerobic Training

Four to six times a week, you'll do twenty minutes of aerobic activity (either after your resistance training or on the days in between). Warm up for five minutes at a low intensity, then perform twenty minutes of aerobic activity within your target heart rate zone. Cool down with five more minutes at a low intensity.

Resistance Training

Warm-up with a low-intensity activity for five minutes, then perform each Lucky Thirteen move in the order given, resting 60 to 180 seconds between each set.

When to Change

Stick with this program for three to four weeks. Afterward, substitute each of the Lucky Thirteen exercises you've been using for another variation.

MONDAYS
(Legs workout)

The Lucky Thirteen Move	The Type of Move You Should Use	How Many Sets?	How Many Reps?
Squat	Primary only	4	8–10
Squat	Primary or secondary	3	8–10
Squat	Primary or secondary	3	8–10
Lunge	Primary only	3	8–10
Lunge	Primary or secondary	3	8–10
Lunge	Primary or secondary	3	8–10
Crunch	Primary only	2–3	10–15
Reverse crunch	Primary only	2–3	10–15
		TOTAL SETS 23–25	

TUESDAYS
(Chest workout)

The Lucky Thirteen Move	The Type of Move You Should Use	How Many Sets?	How Many Reps?
Chest press	Primary only	4	8–10
Chest press	Primary or secondary	4	8–10
Chest press	Primary or secondary	3	8–10
Chest fly	Primary only	3	8–10
Chest fly	Primary or secondary	3	8–10
Crunch	Primary or secondary	2–3	10–15
Reverse crunch	Primary only	2–3	10–15
		TOTAL SETS 21–23	

WEDNESDAYS
(Back workout)

The Lucky Thirteen Move	The Type of Move You Should Use	How Many Sets?	How Many Reps?
Row	Primary only	4	8–10
Row	Primary or secondary	3	8–10
Row	Primary or secondary	3	8–10
Pulldown	Primary only	3	8–10
Pulldown	Primary or secondary	3	8–10
Pulldown	Primary or secondary	3	8–10
Crunch	Primary only	2–3	10–15
Reverse crunch	Primary only	2–3	10–15
		TOTAL SETS 23–25	

THURSDAYS
(Shoulder workout)

The Lucky Thirteen Move	The Type of Move You Should Use	How Many Sets?	How Many Reps?
Shoulder press	Primary only	4	8–10
Shoulder press	Primary or secondary	4	8–10
Raise	Primary only	3	8–10
Raise	Primary or secondary	3	8–10
Raise	Primary or secondary	3	8–10
Crunch	Primary only	2–3	10–15
Reverse crunch	Primary only	2–3	10–15
		TOTAL SETS 21–23	

FRIDAYS
(Biceps workout)

The Lucky Thirteen Move	The Type of Move You Should Use	How Many Sets?	How Many Reps?
Curl	Primary only	4	8–10
Curl	Primary or secondary	4	8–10
Curl	Primary or secondary	4	8–10
Crunch	Primary only	2–3	10–15
Reverse crunch	Primary only	2–3	10–15
		TOTAL SETS 16–18	

SATURDAYS
(Triceps workout)

The Lucky Thirteen Move	The Type of Move You Should Use	How Many Sets?	How Many Reps?
Pressdown	Primary only	4	8–10
Pressdown	Primary or secondary	4	8–10
Extension	Primary only	4	8–10
Extension	Primary or secondary	4	8–10
Crunch	Primary only	2–3	10–15
Reverse crunch	Primary only	2–3	10–15
	TOTAL SETS 20–22		

Superstars and Super People

Let me leave you with a couple of quick anecdotes of clients that I have been lucky enough to work out with over the years. These are not Heisman Trophy winners, not NBA champions, not Stanley Cup winners, not tennis Grand-Slam winners, not heavyweight champions or welterweight champions of the world. They are not action heroes, not models, not Oscar winners, not Emmy winners, and not Grammy winners. These are people who had their own goals and concerns, as real as rain in their world certainly as real as anyone else's—just as real as your goals. Each person's concerns and goals are as valid as the next. Some worry about getting camera-ready for the red carpet, some worry about their upcoming high school reunion. Some find motivation by thinking about the nude scene they will have to film in a few weeks, some find motivation thinking about the family Hawaiian vacation. Some get pumped for a championship bout, some for the eighty-two-plus-game NBA season. Some are even closer to home than these. Listen up . . .

I had a forty-four-year old lady who asked me to teach her how to rollerblade so that she could do more with her nine-year-old daughter. I trained a fifty-something-year-old guy, who was lying on the floor of his home gym in the fetal position when I showed up one day because he said he was just too tired to do *anything* anymore. He was HIV positive and had been for nearly ten years. Sometimes he didn't leave his house for days. I started taking him on outdoor walks for the second half of his workouts and kept his resistance training varied, fun, and challenging. He put on about twelve pounds over the course of the next two years while we worked out. He went to Europe, India, and Japan during that time and started training with me at a private gym instead of his home, even though he had originally told one that he'd never go to a gym.

I had a guy who was a Harvard Law School graduate who was in his mid-thirties, beyond successful from an outsider's point of view. During one workout, he turned to me and asked if I would help teach him how to walk. He felt as though his walk was funny (it wasn't, for a Canada goose) and said that it made it tough to get a girl friend. I did help him, which was one of the more hilarious experiences of my career, and he got a girlfriend. I don't believe the two were connected, but he did, and he was happy. Job well done in my book. Just goes to show what a little added confidence can do for a person. Or a Canada goose.

I had a man bring his ninety, yes, *ninety*-year-old sister to me because she wasn't active enough and suffered from dementia. He felt that working out would help her and that my sense of humor would keep her "in the moment." She would ask me during our workouts if I were still the president (I was, but just of the gym, not the country) and how I liked Washington. *Just fine thank you*, I'd reply without ever having left Los Angeles. She became more alert and focused over time, and she realized that I was not the president, but just a diplomatic young man who wanted her to feel good and get the most out of every day.

Her brother called me about a year after they had moved and told me that she had passed away but that what we had done, the three of us, by getting her in the gym and into a routine, had made her life infinitely better and that she had asked after me regularly when they left LA. I think she even supported my reelection.

My point here is that these people, and many others, stepped into fitness with very different goals and reasons for these goals. The common denominator in what they achieved was a new lease on life. They all went on to participate in their lives. Before long, they found themselves doing things they had previously written off as impossible. Many of them reached new personal highs. They were all successful people, experiencing fresh success because they had a fresh purpose.

Helping them, I have been constantly reminded of my own transformation from a fat kid to a fitness guy and the incredible sense of accomplishment it has brought me. And I've realized how much power finding the right purpose can have over the rest of your life—at any time in your life. Plus, it feels great winning a couple of rounds in the fight against time.

It all starts now.

So get to it!

NOTES

NOTES

NOTES

NOTES

NOTES

NOTES

NOTES

NOTES